Drawing the Line on

Calories, Carbs, and Fat

Connect-the-Dots Approach to Good Health!

Roberta Schwartz Wennik, M.S., R.D.N.

Labyrinth Publishing Works

Labyrinth Publishing Works
P.O. Box 83
Lynnwood, Washington 98046-0083

ISBN 978-0-9623055-3-5

10 9 8 7 6 5 4 3 2 1

DRAWING THE LINE

Contents

Introduction

Welcome to *Drawing the Line on Calories, Carbs, and Fat,* the unique patented system that is going to make tracking calories, carbohydrates and fat quick and easy to do. Research shows that people who monitor what they eat have the best weight-loss results, along with achieving better eating habits. That's because paying attention to what you're eating, especially by the "drawing-the-line" approach, helps keep you focused on what's working and what isn't.

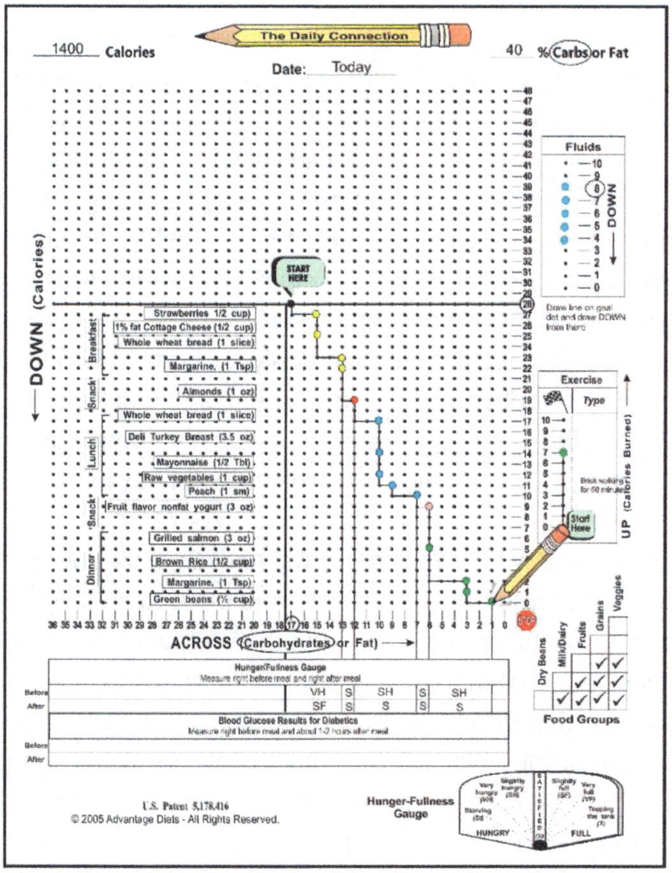

This system got its name from what you'll be doing to keep track of your nutrient intake — that is, "drawing the line" across a matrix of dots on "The Daily Connection". You literally create a picture of what you eat. Maybe you remember as a child connecting dots in a book to make the picture of a horse or maybe a hot air balloon. Now you'll be doing it for a day's intake of food. Hearing that a food contains 500 calories may sound like a lot of calories (or maybe not), but seeing it drawn out on paper in relation to your day's allowance is an eye-opening experience. It may make you think twice about your food choices. This is nothing like you've ever tried before. Yet, after trying it, you'll probably find that it's the best thing you ever did for yourself in your efforts to lose weight and become healthier.

I've provided you with a blank template of *The Daily Connection* in the Appendix that you can make copies of. I also have a print book of *Daily Connections* called "Drawing the Line on Calories, Carbs, and Fat — *Daily Connections"* that you can buy on Amazon. You may find it more convenient. It contains 100 of these templates.

As you also will see in the Appendix, there are Food Lists sorted in various ways to make *drawing the line* easy for you. I'll be talking about them in a moment. The most effective way to use this system is to do it at the time you're eating. Therefore, in order to have the Food Lists available at such time, not only are the Food Lists at the end of this book, there is an electronic book available called "Drawing the Line on Calories, Carbs, and Fat — *Food Lists*" that you can get on Amazon and download to your cell phone or electronic device. That way you'll always have the Food Lists with you.

Let me just say again, the idea about tracking what you're eating is not to track it after you've eaten it, but check before you eat to see how much you have to spend on calories, carbohydrates, and fat. Otherwise, you'll probably find you've gone over your allowances for each nutrient.

If you like the idea of tracking your food intake on the computer or an electronic device (tablet or cell phone), you could do one of the following after printing out a copy of *The Daily Connection.* First, follow the instructions in Chapter 2 – Getting Started to set up a personal *Daily Connection* tailored to your needs, drawing in the start lines (as you see in the example above). Then,

- Scan it into your computer as a Word document. Using the "Insert Shapes" tool in Word, you can actually "draw the line" electronically on *The Daily Connection*.
- Or, take a picture of *The Daily Connection* on your phone or tablet. Then, use the text tool in your picture edit function to "draw the line".

Just find the way that works best for you because something you don't use won't be of any help to you.

A recommendation: Before you make any changes to the way you're eating, talk with your doctor first about what changes you plan to make just to be sure they're the right changes for you personally. That's especially true for those who have diabetes. Consult your healthcare provider, dietitian and/or certified diabetes educator to coordinate what you eat with any diabetes medication you may be taking. You may want to take a copy of *The Daily Connection* with you to share with your healthcare provider or dietitian to have them help set eating goals for you. This approach is not intended as a substitute for medical advice, but as a wonderful addition to your health and/or weight-loss management.

With this connect-the-dots approach, you'll definitely **see** on paper and on your body how calories count! Eat too many of them, whether in the form of carbohydrates, fat or protein, and you'll gain weight. The question is, "Which nutrient should you eat less of?" Should you take a Low-Carb approach**,** a Low-Fat approach or maybe just a Balanced approach to eating? By the way, all approaches work as long as you stick to it.

You get to choose what appeals to you and works for you. Want to try the *Low-Carb* diet because you've heard it's a fairly easy way to lose weight, or maybe you have diabetes and need to control the amount of carbohydrates you eat? *Drawing the Line* is a fun way to do it. (By the way, while I may refer to these various approaches as "diets", I don't want you to think, as most people do, that diet = restriction. You can choose whatever foods you want that fit on *The Daily Connection.*) Or maybe you think that eating too much fat has led to your weight problem, or you have high cholesterol and should be following a *Low-Fat* approach. You can do that with *Drawing the Line,* as well. If you don't like the idea of drastically cutting either carbohydrates or fat, then take the *Balanced* approach.

You might even consider rotating between the different approaches, especially when you hit a plateau, where it seems like nothing you do helps you lose any more weight. Maybe you've reached your goal weight, but have started to gain it back. You shouldn't worry about gaining back a couple of pounds since one's weight can fluctuate from day to day. But you should set 3 to 5 pounds as your limit for fluctuation. If that happens, then "draw the line" for a week or so as a refresher course.

This innovative system gives you the flexibility to tailor your weight-loss and health efforts to what you personally need. To help you with your decision, here's some information about each type of diet.

The Low-Carb Diet

People can lose weight on a low-carb diet, partly because it's both a low-calorie diet and higher-protein diet. The major benefit people find with the low-carb diet is that they're able to control their hunger better even though they're eating less food. The increased amount of protein is more satisfying and satiating than the carbohydrates it replaces.

If you try the low-carb diet, it would be a good idea to take a general vitamin and mineral supplement. Also, keep in mind that you'll need to select your proteins wisely to avoid eating too much saturated fat. (Healthy food selections will be covered a little later in the book.)

Drawing the Line allows you to eat as little as 35% of your calories from carbohydrates, an amount that is low but not extreme. However, starting at 40 to 45% of total calories would help you wean yourself off of carbohydrates and give you a chance to see if this is the right approach for you. You might want to move toward the Balanced diet as you approach your goal weight or when you find that the approach you've chosen is no longer as effective. With *Drawing the Line*, you can gradually add more carbs back into your diet in a controlled way—a way that will help you avoid regaining the lost pounds. In a few moments I'll show you how you can set the level of nutrients you should be eating.

Who Should Be on a Low-Carb Diet?

The low-carb diet can be effective for many different people. If you've struggled with getting the weight off and need to become motivated again, the low-carb diet will produce a fairly rapid weight loss, at first, *without* the usual hunger associated with dieting. If you have high triglycerides, a decrease in carbohydrates would help lower that level.

If you have diabetes, especially if you're on insulin, you have to control the amount of carbohydrates you eat at any one time. If you don't, you will tend to get spikes in your blood sugar level, making it very difficult for your body to bring the level back into an acceptable range. *Drawing the Line* makes it possible to match the amount of insulin diabetics give themselves with the amount of carbohydrates they eat—because tracking or *counting carbohydrates* is so easy. If you have diabetes, you should speak with your healthcare provider, dietitian or diabetes educator to help you determine what percentage of calories should come from carbohydrates. Take a copy of *The Daily Connection* with you to share with them how you plan to track your carb intake.

The Low-Fat Diet

It would seem to make sense that if you're overweight and carrying around too much extra body fat, you should eliminate some fat from your diet, especially considering that a gram of fat has twice as many calories as a gram of carbohydrate or protein. (Of course, just remember that too much of any nutrient can lead to excess body fat.)

Food manufacturers have been more than helpful in providing low-fat and non-fat foods. However, people have mistakenly believed they can eat as much as they want of these foods—forgetting that *calories count*. In addition, many of these low- and non-fat foods have replaced fat with sugar. Talk about being counterproductive. While packaged foods that are low in fat can be handy occasionally, better to focus on the foods that are *naturally* low in fat, such as fruits, vegetables and whole grains. (In most cases, they're also less expensive.) In fact, a truly low-fat diet is quite high in "good" carbohydrates—complex starches—rather than the refined carbohydrates found in sugar and white flour, baked goods and sweets.

If you can't imagine giving up carbohydrates (like a delicious sourdough bread or artisan wheat bread), then a low-fat diet may be right for you. Also, you have to be ever vigilant to food labels to see just how much sugar replaced the fat.

Consider "grazing" your way through the day by eating three meals and two to three snacks to avoid feeling hungry. Also, remember to choose your carbohydrates wisely, opting for complex carbs such as dry beans, whole grains, fruits and vegetables.

Even though *Drawing the Line* allows you to track as little as 10% of your calories from fat, it is suggested that you start with a 20% to 25% level first. If you've been eating closer to the American average of 40% of your calories from fat, it will be easier to gradually work your way down. Unfortunately, for many much of that 40% is made up of unhealthy saturated fats. As with the other two types of approaches, you can set the percentage level of nutrients you want to eat. Just remember to make your fat choices healthy fats (e.g. olive oil, walnuts, canola oil).

Who Should Be on a Low-Fat Diet?

People with heart disease, high blood pressure, high cholesterol, or who have a family history of these diseases, should be on either a low-fat diet or a balanced diet. While they could be on a low-carb diet, careful selection of protein would be necessary to avoid too much fat. Cutting back on fat (especially saturated fat) helps to decrease the level of LDL-cholesterol (the bad cholesterol in the blood). Selecting healthier fats can help increase the level of HDL-cholesterol (the good cholesterol). You'll read more about these fats a little later in the book.

Because a low-fat diet tends to be higher in fruits, vegetables and whole grains, people with certain types of cancer may benefit from the higher levels of antioxidants found in this kind of diet. As with the low-carb diet, a low-fat diet also works well for people who need to lose weight. Not only is fat decreased, but the amount of food allowed is greater. And if higher fiber foods are selected, there is greater appetite suppression and hunger satiation.

The Balanced Diet

A balanced diet is really the most sensible diet of all. That's because you're balancing the percentages of total calories coming from carbohydrates, fat and protein so that no one nutrient dominates your diet. There have been numerous diets through the years suggesting various combinations of these percentages. The traditional mix used to be 55-65% carbohydrates, 30% fat and 15% protein. At that time, it was thought that carbohydrates and fat were the most effective at satisfying hunger. Yet, recent studies are showing that protein probably keeps hunger at bay the longest.

Drawing the Line makes it possible for you to try a variety of combinations to determine what works best for you. You might start with a mix of 45% carbs, 25% protein, and 30% fat. This should provide enough protein to deal with your hunger and with a high enough level of carbs to get the necessary vitamins, minerals and fiber.

For a diet to be sensible (and it really should be when it's something that hopefully you'll follow the rest of your life), you have to be smart in your food choices. A little later in the book you'll read about healthy food choices, but one major objective with a balanced diet is trying to eat more foods that are less processed. By doing so, you'll decrease the amount of sodium and sugar you're eating, since these are two main ingredients found in many processed foods. You'll also be eating foods in their more natural state, taking advantage of the bounty and balance of nutrients they naturally contain.

Who Should Be on a Balanced Diet?

Almost anyone can be on balanced diet, whether you have weight to lose or not. If you can't see yourself giving up carbs or forsaking the flavor of fat, a balanced diet may be right for you. The tracking done with *Drawing the Line* is the same for all three types of diets. The only difference are the levels of nutrients monitored.

CHAPTER 1

A Sneak Preview

The Daily Connection is the chart on which you'll be tracking the foods you eat. You'll be monitoring two nutrients at a time. No matter whether you're following the Low-Carb Diet, Low-Fat Diet, or the Balanced Diet, *calories* will always be one of the measurements. It can't be said often enough that "calories count!" When you're on the Low-Carb Diet you'll be tracking carbohydrates as the second nutrient. On the Low-Fat and the Balanced Diets, you'll monitor fat as the second nutrient.

Let's look at a completed *Daily Connection* to see how it works. (See Figure 1 on the next page.) This sample *Daily Connection* is set up for a woman named Linda who is following the Low-Carb diet, eating 1400 calories a day, with 40% of those calories coming from carbohydrates. (Notice that she circled the word "Carbs" at the top and bottom of the *Daily Connection* just as a reminder for herself.) Fortunately, *Drawing the Line* is so flexible that Linda can continue to make adjustments as she sees fit. Fewer calories? No problem. More carbs? No problem. All she need do is adjust her horizontal and vertical lines as you will soon see.

There are so many things you can track on *The Daily Connection:* your hunger level, amount of fluid you drink per day, the time devoted to exercise, what food groups you've eaten from. For people who have diabetes, you can even log in your blood sugar numbers before and after eating. The nice part is that you don't have to do them all. Just choose the sections that you're most interested in. I'll be describing them in detail in just a moment. You may want to try a section for a short while to determine if it's something you want to track. Then add another section, again deciding if it's of value to you. You're free to use all or just some of the parts of *The Daily Connection.* Just realize that the more involved you get with *The Daily Connection*, the greater your success will be.

Think "Down-and-Across"

Remember, Linda is on the *Low-Carb* diet. So, every time Linda eats something, she draws a line DOWN through a certain number of dots for the calories in the food and then ACROSS for the amount of carbohydrates in the food. (Had she been on the Low-Fat or Balanced Diet, then the ACROSS numbers would be for fat.) The number of dots can be found either in the Food Lists (found in the Appendix) or can be determined from information found on packaged food labels (I'll share with you what to look for and how to use the information very soon). For each food she eats, she basically draws the line "DOWN-and-ACROSS". What could be easier?

Looking at *The Daily Connection* below, you can see that Linda's breakfast consists of cottage cheese topped with strawberries. She also had a slice of whole wheat toast spread with margarine. Figure 2 shows you an excerpted version of the Food List that helped Linda determine how many dots to draw her line through. Under FRUITS, she found strawberries are worth "1 DOWN" for the calories and "2 ACROSS" for the carbs. Go back to Figure 1 to see how she drew the line DOWN 1-and-ACROSS 2 for the strawberries. Under CHEESE, she finds that cottage cheese has "2 DOWN" for calories and "0 ACROSS" for carbs (no appreciable amount of carbohydrates). Under BREAD, whole wheat toast is worth "2 DOWN" for calories and "2 ACROSS" for carbs. Note that Linda only had 1 teaspoon of margarine, so she divided the margarine listed (1 tablespoon) in half for easy drawing — "1 DOWN" and "0 ACOSS". She continues doing the same process for all the foods she eats for the remainder of the day.

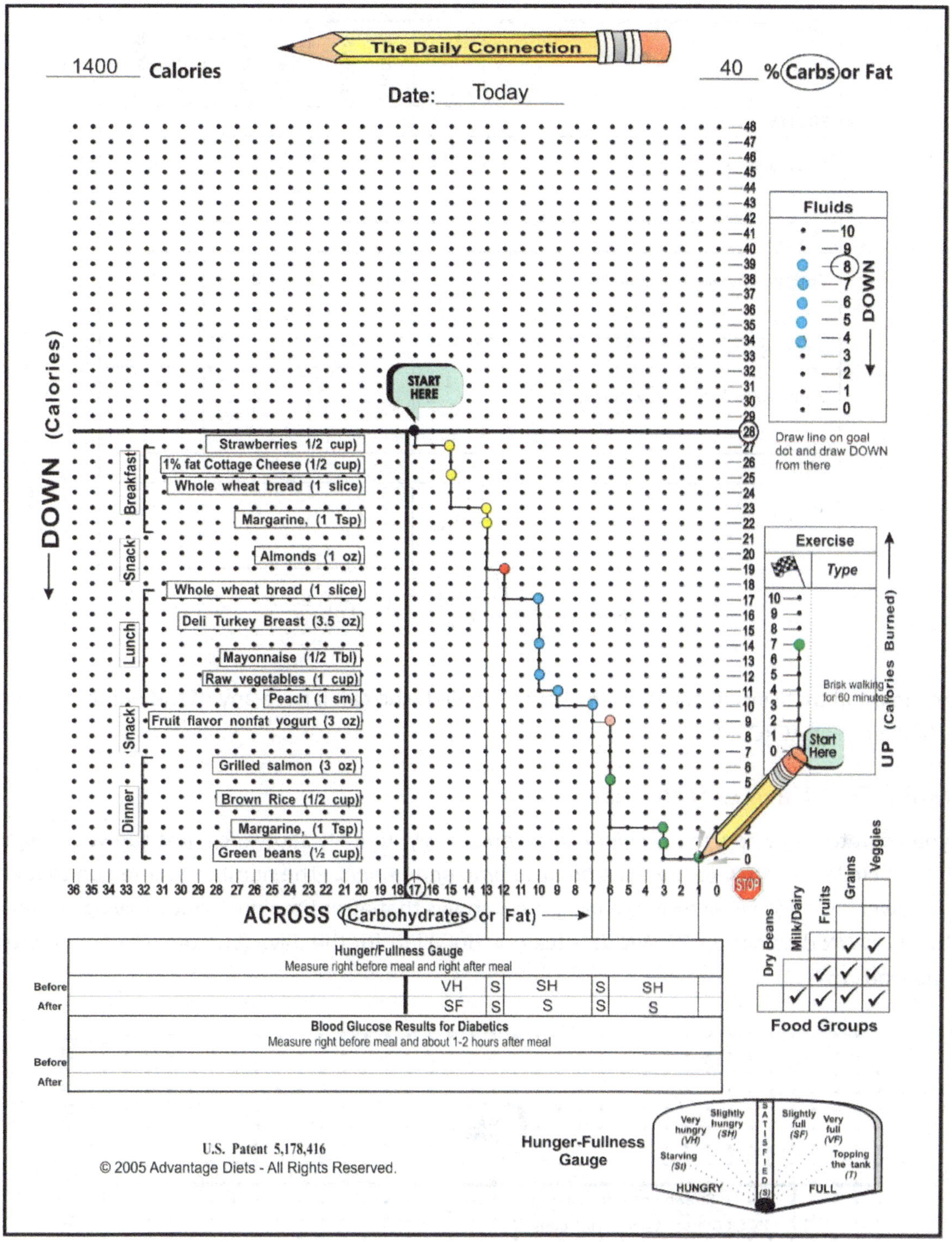

Figure 1

Example of The Daily Connection — 1400 Calories and 40% Carbohydrates

ALPHABETICAL				
FOOD	Amt	Calories DOWN	Carbs ACROSS	Fat ACROSS
FRUITS				
Strawberries ...	½ cup	1	2	0
CHEESE				
Cottage Cheese, Low Fat 1% ...	½ cup	2	0	0
BREADS				
Bread - whole wheat, whole grain ...	1 slice	2	2	0
FATS				
Margarine ...	1 tbsp	2	0	4

Figure 2
Sample Entries from the Food List

Keep in mind that since Linda is on the Low-Carb diet, she can ignore any of the numbers in the column labeled "Fat ACROSS").

How Much Do I Have Left to Eat?

When you want to know how many *calorie dots* remain in your daily allowance, just run your finger across from the last circle you drew to the *right-hand column of numbers.* The number you see on that line tells you the answer. The following example in Figure 3 shows that after breakfast, Riley having started the day out with 24 DOWN dots had 17 DOWN dots (calorie dots) left for the day. (See the number where the green line leads to?)

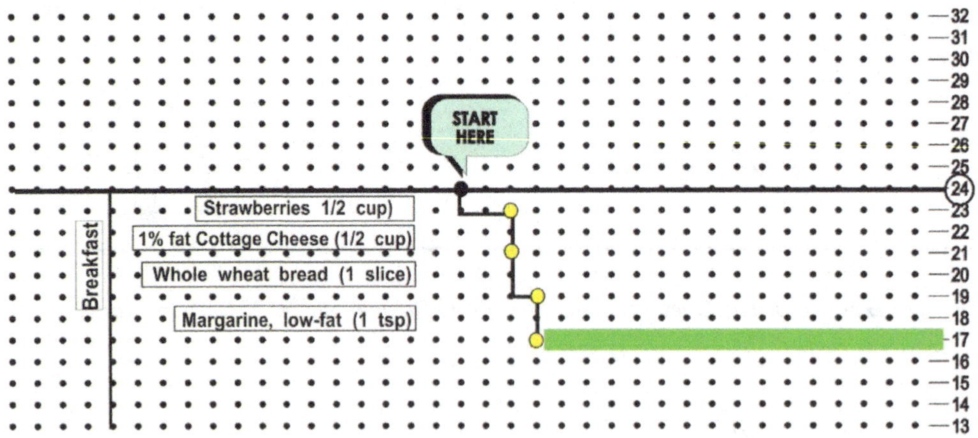

Figure 3
Number of DOWN Dots Remaining After Breakfast

You also can see how many more ACROSS dots (in this case, carbohydrates) Riley had remaining after breakfast by *looking to the numbers at the bottom* of *The Daily Connection* from that same last circle. Check out where the blue line leads in Figure 4. In this case, there are 15 ACROSS dots (carbohydrate dots) left after breakfast.

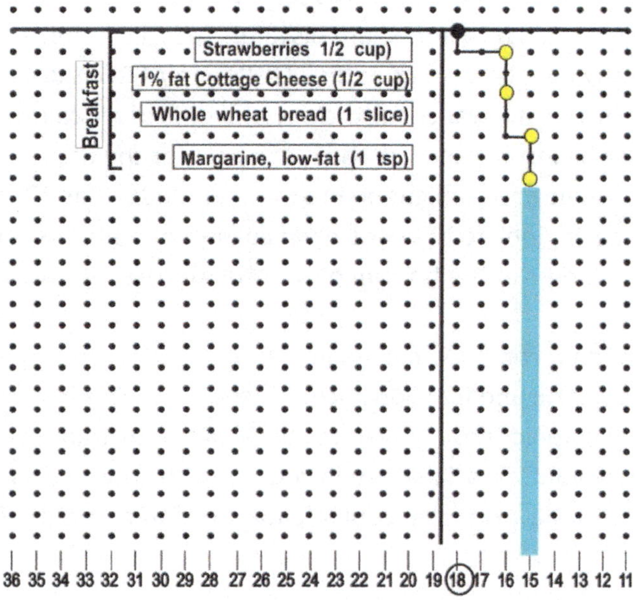

Figure 4
Number of ACROSS Dots Remaining After Breakfast

Let's face it. If you had a bank account with $500 in it, you couldn't go spending $850. The bank would stop payment. The same should go for your nutrient account. There's only so much in it to spend during the day. Look at it on the bright side—at least your "nutrient" accounts (i.e., calories, carbs, and fat) are replenished every day. Now don't you wish your bank would do that for you?

While Riley had wanted to have lasagna for dinner, she did the right thing. She first checked to see how many DOWN and ACROSS dots she had remaining, looking to the numbers on the right and the numbers on the bottom of *The Daily Connection.* After checking the DOWN and ACROSS numbers in the Food List for lasagna, she realized she didn't have enough DOWN dots for lasagna today. She opted for a grilled chicken breast instead. If she wants lasagna tomorrow, she'll just choose different foods during the day that will allow her to have enough dots for the lasagna. That's being proactive and smart. Good for you, Riley!

Most people shy away from keeping traditional food diaries because it requires a lot of math. As an example, that of keeping track of the number of calories you've eaten: First you have to add the number of calories for the meal. Then you have to subtract that number from the daily allowance. That works great for breakfast, but now for all the other foods you eat, you'll have to keep a running balance to subtract the calorie values from for the next food you eat and each food you eat. And that's just for calories. With *Drawing the Line,* there's no math to do. This patented system takes care of that for you! That's what those blue and green lines we just saw are all about.

A Picture Is Worth a Thousand Words

The beauty of *Drawing the Line* is how graphic it is. Depending upon what you eat, the picture you draw can be very enlightening. Let's take Joe as an example, who's on a Balanced Diet, eating 1800 calories a day, with 30% of his calories coming from fat. After a reasonable breakfast, he decided to eat at McDonald's for lunch, ordering a Big Mac®, medium French fries, and a 16-ounce serving of soda. *The Daily Connection* on the next page (Figure 5) shows Joe's breakfast and lunch so far for the day.

As it turns out, Joe drew the line **after** he ate his lunch (not a recommended way to use this system). Notice the yellow square showing how much of his DOWN and ACROSS dots he used up just for lunch. That's a whopping 78% of his fat allowance for the day and 47% of his calorie allowance. It's only after he drew the line did he realize he left himself with next to no fat for the day. It looks like a dinner of vegetables, legumes, and whole grains might be in order. While Joe has 12 DOWN dots worth of calories left to spend for the day (again, look to the right-hand column of numbers), he has only 2 ACROSS dots worth of fat (look to the numbers at the bottom of the sheet). The red square shows how little fat he can have for dinner.

Until using *The Daily Connection,* Joe had no idea that a McDonald lunch could take such a big bite (pun intended!) out of his calorie and fat allowances for the day. This is where *Drawing the Line* becomes so valuable. You get a real graphic sense of how many calories and grams of fat or carbohydrates (depending upon which one you're tracking) are in your food. It truly shows how you've spent your allowances for the day. With this example, wouldn't you say that a "picture *is* worth a thousand words?"

Advantages of the Different Food Lists

Using Joe's mistake as an example, it becomes clear that learning to become *proactive* is critical. Eating something and *then* drawing the line for it (a reactive approach), makes it too easy to go over your daily nutrient allowance. *Drawing the Line* gives you a way to know whether a food choice will work for you. You select your foods based on your available dots so you don't run out. Instead of Joe having had the Big Mac®, medium French fries and the soda, which cost him a total of 18 DOWN dots and 18 ACROSS dots, he could have selected a Cheeseburger, a small order of French fries, and a diet soda—spending 11 DOWN dots and 9 ACROSS dots. Then he would have left himself with 18 DOWN dots of calories (instead of 12) for the remainder of the day and 11 ACROSS dots of fat (instead of 2), enough to have even had an afternoon snack.

The idea is not to have to give up everything you enjoy but select foods that you like that will fit into your overall intake for the day. *Drawing the Line* has four different *Food Lists* to help you out. First, there is an Alphabetical listing. If you know what food you want to eat, look it up under its food category and then find it alphabetically.

In times when you're looking for foods with a certain number of dots to allow you to stay within your daily allowance, there are three other lists sorted as "least to most". Maybe you're trying to find something with the least number of calories. Then you look at the Food List that is sorted from "Least to Most Calories". The same thing applies to the "Least to Most Carbs" and the "Least to Most Fat". Check them out in the Appendix.

By the way, don't forget to take note of the quantity of food ("Amt" column) in the *Food List.* If you have more than that, it needs to be accounted for.

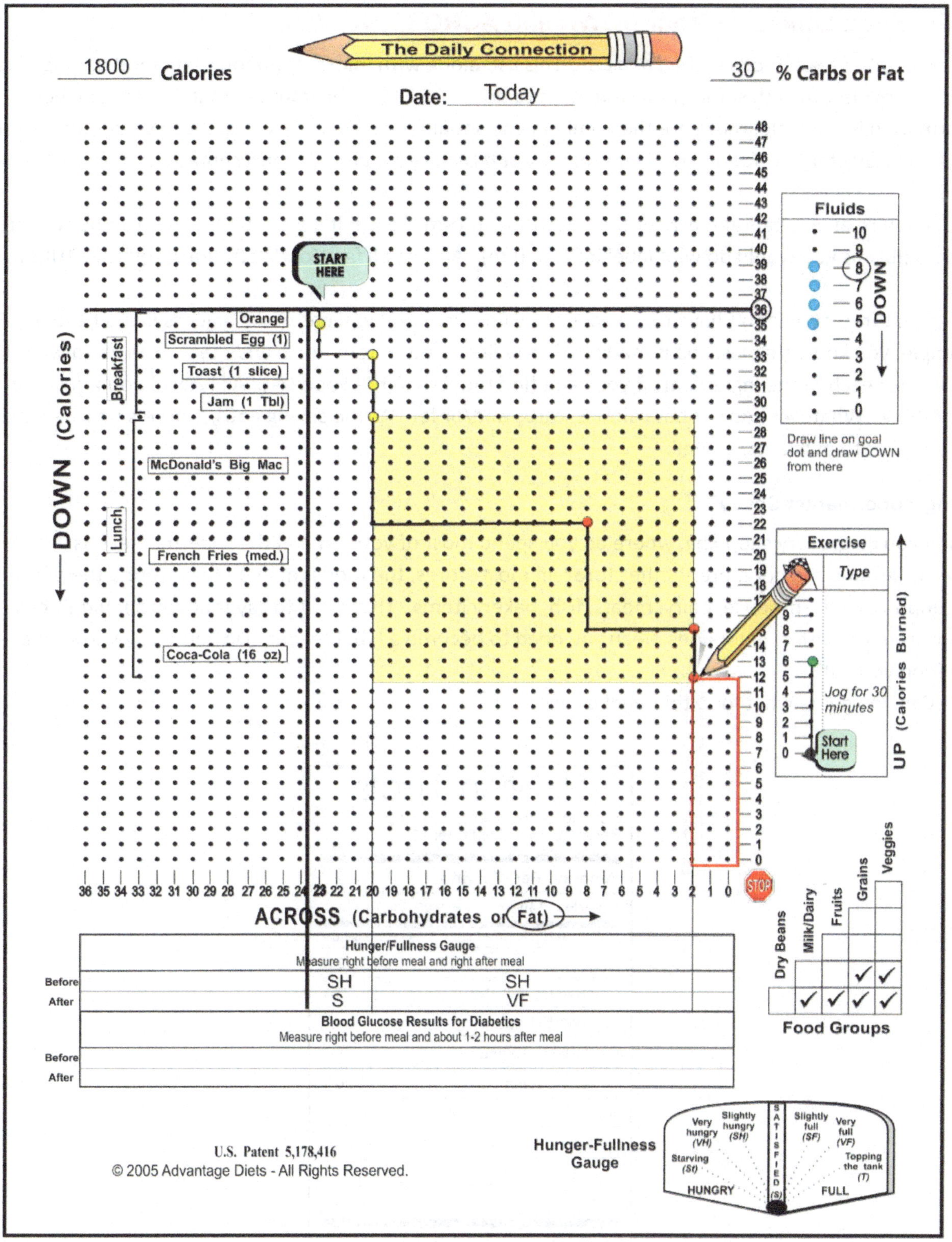

Figure 5

Joe's Daily Connection Having Had Lunch at McDonald's

Using Food Labels for Your DOWN and ACROSS Numbers

There are about 800 foods in the *Food List*. This list, along with information found on food package labels, should provide you with sufficient information to *draw the line.* I recommend that whenever label information is available, those are the numbers you should use. That's because those values on the label are specifically for that food. The values in the *Food List* are for generic representations of a particular food.

If you're at a restaurant, ask for their nutrition information (if it's available). It too can be converted to dots (just as you would do with label information). Almost all fast-food restaurants offer Nutrition Facts.

Don't fret if you don't have the exact details for each food you eat. Take a guess if you have to. For example, you know that lasagna is made with noodles, cheese, tomatoes, and meat. You can always *draw the line* for each of the ingredients if you can't find the dish in the Food List. All I ask of you is just log something. Whatever you eat has calories, carbs and/or fat. As the saying goes, "there's no free lunch". That applies to nutrients, as well.

Being Supermarket Savvy

When you go grocery shopping, where do you spend most of your time in the supermarket? Is it in the aisles or around the perimeter of the store? In most stores, the foods that you find around the perimeter are unprocessed—produce, dairy, meats, fish, bakery items. That's not to say that you shouldn't buy foods from the aisles, but it does mean you need to become a label reader. Do you really know what's in the food you eat?

Can you guess what food this label is for?

Nutrition Facts

Serving Size ½ cup (130 g)
Servings Per Container 6

Amount Per Serving	
Calories 140	Calories from Fat 10
	% Daily Value*
Total Fat 1g	2%
Saturated Fat 0g	0%
Trans Fat 0g	
Cholesterol 130mg	0%
Sodium 620mg	26%
Total Carbohydrate 28g	7%
Dietary Fiber 5g	20%
Sugars 11g	
Protein 6g	

Vitamin A	0%	•	Vitamin C	2%
Calcium	6%	•	Iron	10%

INGREDIENTS: WATER, PREPARED WHITE BEANS, SUGAR, MUSTARD, (VINEGAR, WATER, MUSTARD SEED, SALT, NATURAL FLAVOR), MAPLE CURED BACON, SALT, PURE MAPLE SYRUP, CORN STARCH, ONION POWDER, CARAMEL COLOR, TAPIOCA MALTODEXTRIN, AUTOLYZED YEAST EXTRACT, BACON FAT, NATURAL FLAVORS AND NATURAL SMOKE FLAVOR.

Before you find out what the food is, would you say that it's a healthy choice? It's definitely a low-fat food. And it's especially good because it doesn't have any saturated or *trans* fat — *trans* fat being even worse for you than saturated fat. Both contribute to high cholesterol. The sodium in this food is a bit high for a food that contains 140 calories.

> A Rule of Thumb: The milligrams of sodium should be no more than 1 to 1½ times the total number of calories (in this case, it should be about 140-210 mg of sodium per serving rather than 620 mg).

Even so, this food is a good source of protein.

Also notice that, under the "Total Carbohydrate" section, there's quite a bit of sugar in this food — "Sugars 11 g". That's equivalent to about three teaspoons of sugar per serving. It pays to look at the ingredients on any food you eat. If not only for things like sodium and sugar, but also to make sure that the food doesn't contain anything you might be sensitive to or allergic to. It's especially significant for people who are lactose or gluten intolerant or have celiac disease.

> Important Note: Ingredients are listed in order of most to least weight.

While sugar appears third in the list of ingredients, that's not the only source of sugar. There's also sugar in the maple syrup and maltodextrin, ingredients that appear further down on the list. Clever food manufacturers have figured out how to fool shoppers — whether intentionally or not. By including several different forms of sugar, no single type may have enough weight to put it at the top of the list. But they do add up.

Fortunately, the amount of dietary fiber in this food is impressive. With 5 grams of dietary fiber, you're getting about 15-25% of the 20-38 grams of fiber you should be eating per day. Fiber helps to control swings in blood glucose, by slowing down the digestion process and allowing smaller amounts of glucose to enter the bloodstream at one time. It helps keep you off the rollercoaster of high energy to lethargy. This is especially helpful for people with diabetes. Also, fiber serves as a great probiotic for gut bacteria. Happy gut bacteria make for a healthier person.

The recommended daily intake of total fiber set by the government for adults 50 years and younger is 38 grams for men and 25 grams for women. For men and women over 50, it's 30 and 21 grams, respectively.

So, have you figured out what food this label is for? It's Baked Beans.

How to Track Food Label Info on *The Daily Connection*

In order to make label information easy to use on *The Daily Connection*, the following table (Table 7) is indispensable. The first section shows you how to convert the **Calories** on the label to **DOWN** dots; the second section is for converting **Total Carbohydrates** shown on the label to **ACROSS** dots and the last section is for converting **Total Fat** shown on the label to **ACROSS** dots. Again, whether you track carbohydrates or fat depends upon what type of diet you're following.

CALORIES				TOTAL CARBS				TOTAL FAT			
The label shows Calories to be:			DOWN	The label shows Total Carbs to be:			ACROSS	The label shows Total Fat to be:			ACROSS
1	to	24	0	1	to	4	0	0	to	1	0
25	to	74	1	5	to	12	1	2	to	3	1
75	to	124	2	13	to	20	2	4	to	6	2
125	to	174	3	21	to	29	3	7	to	9	3
175	to	224	4	30	to	37	4	10	to	11	4
225	to	274	5	38	to	46	5	12	to	14	5
275	to	324	6	47	to	54	6	15	to	16	6
325	to	374	7	55	to	62	7	17	to	19	7
375	to	424	8	63	to	71	8	20	to	22	8
425	to	474	9	72	to	79	9	23	to	24	9
475	to	524	10	80	to	88	10	25	to	27	10
525	to	574	11	89	to	96	11	28	to	29	11
575	to	624	12	97	to	104	12	30	to	32	12
625	to	674	13	105	to	113	13	33	to	34	13
675	to	724	14	114	to	121	14	35	to	37	14
725	to	774	15	122	to	130	15	38	to	40	15
775	to	824	16	131	to	138	16	41	to	42	16
825	to	874	17	139	to	146	17	43	to	45	17

Table 1
Food Label Conversion Table

Tracking the Baked Beans on *The Daily Connection* Using the Conversion table.

For Calories:
From the label information for the Baked Beans above, you can see that a serving contains **140 calories.** Looking at the **CALORIES** section of the conversion table (Table 7), find 140 calories (it's in the row that reads "125 to 174 calories"). It states you should *draw the line* "**DOWN 3 dots**". Okay, now you know that 140 calories are equivalent to 3 DOWN dots.

For Carbohydrates:
For the carbohydrate content of the Baked Beans, look at the "Total Carbohydrate" line on the label. It shows that a serving contains 28 grams. Total Carbohydrates include the starch, sugars and fiber in the baked beans. Looking at the **TOTAL CARBS** section of the conversion table (Table 7), you'll see that 28 grams lands in the 21 to 29 grams row, which is **"ACROSS 3 dots."** That means that 28 grams of carbs is equivalent to 3 ACROSS dots, which, by the way, is merely coincidental with calories being 3 DOWN dots.

If you were on the *Low-Carb Diet,* on *The Daily Connection* you'd be drawing "DOWN 3 dots and ACROSS 3 dots" from the last circle you drew. You would then add another circle after drawing for the Baked Beans.

For Fat:
For the fat content of the Baked Beans, look at the "Total Fat" line on the label. This version of Baked Beans has 1 gram of Total Fat. Looking at Table 7, because Total Fat is so low, you'd have "0 ACROSS". If you were following the *Low-Fat* or *Balanced* diets, in the case of Baked Beans, you would only need to *draw the line* DOWN for the calories.

Even though *Drawing the Line* only requires you to account for the Total Fat in a food, food choice is still important, especially the amount of saturated fat in a food. Saturated fat is problematic because it tends to raise blood cholesterol even more than the cholesterol found in foods (such as in eggs).

> 30% Rule of Thumb for Saturated Fat: Saturated Fat should not be more than 30% of the Total Fat number. Obviously, the Baked Beans are a good choice for both Total Fat and Saturated Fat content. But what if you had a food with a Total Fat content of 15 grams. You'd apply the 30% rule by multiplying 15 grams by .3 = 4.5 grams. If the label states more than 4.5 grams of Saturated Fat for that food, consider finding an alternative food or enjoy it and then select other foods that are lower in saturated fat to make up for it for the remainder of the day.

No matter what packaged food you eat, there will almost always be numbers on the label that you can convert to dots for tracking on *The Daily Connection*. Just use the "Food Label Conversion Table" (Table 7) to help you with the job.

Portion Distortion

As you look at a label, one of the first things you need to check is how much is in a serving. Most of the time, it's much less than what most people would naturally put on their plates. So, I have an assignment for you. Try this experiment, using the Baked Beans as an example. (If you don't normally eat baked beans, choose another canned food and follow this experiment for it.)

1. Without first looking at the label for serving size, serve yourself what you would normally have. Once you have done Steps 2 and 3, come back and measure the amount you served yourself. Write it down.
2. Next, look at the label and find out what a serving size is. Spoon out what you think is that amount on a second plate. After Step 3, come back and measure it. Write it down.
3. On a third plate, measure ½ cup from the can and place it on the plate.

How do your three plates compare? Was what you would normally serve yourself pretty close to what the label stated was a serving size? When you knew how much was in a serving, were you pretty accurate in what you served yourself? If so, good for you and keep up the good work. If not, keep a measuring cup close at hand to continue to practice and learn how to eventually eyeball amounts. That means, don't forget to look at serving sizes on packaged foods.

There will be times when you don't have a measuring cup available. In that case, use the objects in Figure 14 as an aid to measuring various foods. You obviously are not going to be taking a measuring cup with you when you dine out. But that doesn't mean that portion control doesn't apply when you're eating out. *The Daily Connection* does reflect serving amounts.

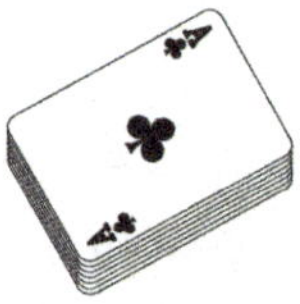

Deck of cards =
3 oz of
cooked meat

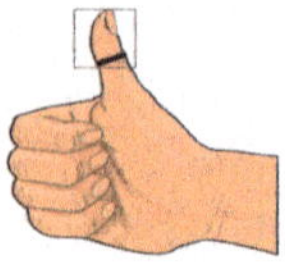

Tip of your thumb =
1 teaspoon

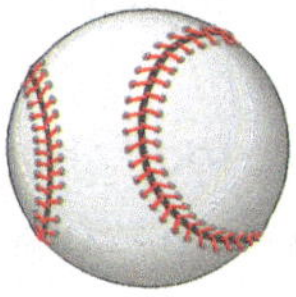

Baseball =
1 cup

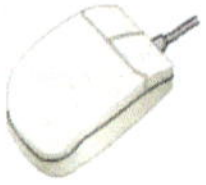

Computer Mouse =
1 potato

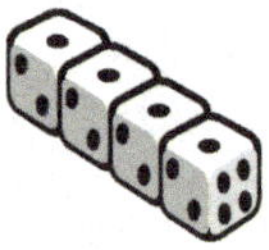

4 Dice =
1 ounce of cheese

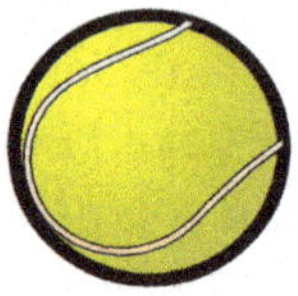

Tennis Ball =
½ cup or
1 medium apple
or peach

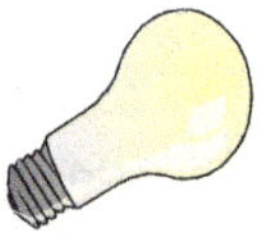

Light bulb =
1 serving of broccoli

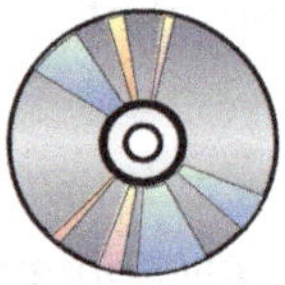

Compact Disc (CD) = 1
pancake

Figure 6
Using Everyday Objects for Portion Control

CHAPTER 2

Getting Started

Hopefully I've teased and tempted you enough by now that you're eager to get started.

Measuring Up

Do you need to lose weight or are you at a healthy weight? Fill in the following blanks to find out.

My height without shoes is ________ inches.

My weight without clothes is __________ pounds. (For consistency, best to weigh yourself in the morning after going to bathroom and wearing no clothes.)

My waist measurement is _____________ inches. (It's best to do this measurement first thing in the morning. Stand up straight without any clothes around your waist. Place the flexible tape measure with the scale facing outward at the smallest point around your middle that's below your rib cage and above your belly button. Don't cinch the tape and don't suck in your gut to get a smaller number. Make sure the tape isn't twisted.)

My hip measurement is ______________ inches. (Your hip measurement should be the widest circle that includes your buttocks. On average, it's about 7 inches below your waist.)

What's Your Waist-to-Hip Ratio?

Divide your waist measurement by your hip measurement.

________	÷	________	=	________
Waist (inches)		Hip (inches)		Ratio

That Ratio will give you an idea what your shape is.

	You are an Apple		You are a Pear
	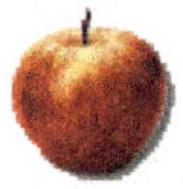	or	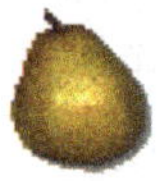
	if your waist-to-hip ratio is:		if your waist-to-hip ratio is:
Women	≥ 0.8		< 0.8
Men	≥ 1.0		< 1.0

You may or may not have heard people talk about their shape in terms of fruits, but there is a reason to know. The shape of your body indicates where you're storing your fat. An apple shape has more fat in the stomach area, while a pear shape carries more of the fat in the hips. Even though women can't stand the idea of having heavy hips, they may be more accepting of being a pear shape when they find out that people who are apple-shaped have a higher risk for Type 2 diabetes, hypertension (high blood pressure) and cardiovascular or heart disease.

A woman's shape is partly due to the effect of her hormones. Pre-menopausal women have high levels of estrogen, which drives the extra fat into the hips and thighs, making their body pear-shaped. Men, on the other hand, have higher levels of testosterone. So they tend to store extra fat in their middle section, giving them the rubber tire or apple look. After menopause, women lose that estrogen advantage. So, as they age, many women start becoming apple-shaped—unless they alter what they eat and how much physical activity they do. Of course, men need to do the same thing to fight their body's natural tendency.

Okay, look at the ratio you got. If you're a woman, is it greater than or equal to 0.8? If so, you'd be considered an apple shape. If you're a man, a ratio of greater than or equal to 1.0 means you're apple-shaped. Another warning number to keep in mind for women is a waist measurement that's greater than 35 inches; in a man, it would be a waist of 40 inches or more.

What's Your BMI?

The initials "BMI" stand for "Body Mass Index." It's a measurement used by most healthcare professionals to determine whether your weight is a healthy one for your height. But, first I want you to determine what your body frame size is. The standard BMI table doesn't take into account your frame size which is a mistake. You could have two people of the same height, one with a small frame and one with a large frame. That large frame consists of more bone mass, which weighs more.

The other thing that is missing from the BMI table that only you personally will know. Athletes tend to be more muscle and less fat than the average person. Runners definitely have less body fat than a weight lifter. Yet, the weight lifter has more muscle than the runner. Then, of course, there's the everyday person who may not be athletic enough to be low in fat and high in muscle. That's more of who the BMI table is accurate for.

Determining Your Frame Size

To figure out your frame size, you'll need a precise measurement of your wrist. Using a flexible tape measure, place it just below that bony protrusion on your wrist. Don't cinch it.

Next, divide your height, in inches, by your wrist measurement, also in inches. The result is your "Frame Size Value".

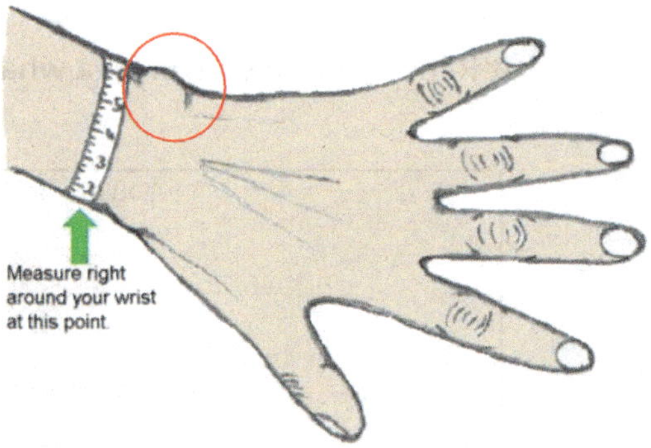

__________ ÷ __________ = __________

Height (inches) Wrist (inches) Frame Size Value

Look at the following table and locate the column for your gender. Then find the Frame Size Value you just calculated. Finally, look to the column at the far right for your frame size. Is that what you thought you were?

FEMALES	MALES	Frame Size Type
Greater than 11.0	Greater than 10.4	Small
10.1 - 11.0	9.6 - 10.4	Medium
Less than 10.1	Less than 9.6	Large

Source: Your Personality Prescription by Roberta Schwartz Wennik, M.S., R.D.

Table 2
Frame Size Values and Types

Using that Frame Size, look at the BMI Table (Table 2 on the next page). Find your height in the leftmost column. Then run your finger across the page until you find the weight you are today. Now look to the top of the chart to find out your BMI number. Write that number here__________ and date it __________.

What section of the table did you end up in? Healthy Weight? Overweight? Obese? Write that here: ______________.

As you can see, that frame size really becomes an issue when you're in the Healthy Weight range. It doesn't come into play when you're overweight or obese since no matter what your frame size, you're still heavier than what is healthy for your height. The BMI gives ranges of weights within each category. Understand that there is not one perfect weight for your height.

Looking at the numbers in the Healthy Weight section of the table for your height, what is your healthy weight range (even if it's not true for you today) when you take into consideration your frame size? Write it here: _______ to _______.

If you're in the Overweight or Obese part of the table, consider setting weight-loss goals that allow you to decrease your weight in steps of 2-3 BMI values. For example, if your BMI is 30, set as your *first* weight-loss goal a BMI of 27 or 28. That certainly should be doable. When you reach that weight, set a new lower BMI goal. Never bite off more than you can chew.

And just remember, weight is just a number, a guidepost. What's more important is considering the health effects of excess weight. No matter how much people don't want to talk about it, weight increases one's risk for heart disease, diabetes, cancer, and a host of other health conditions. And don't forget the effect too much weight has on the joints and one's back. Any weight loss is better than none. Once you start losing weight, you'll actually come to believe you really can. It's like the joke, "How do you eat an elephant?" Answer: One bite at a time.

BODY MASS INDEX 1														
	19	20	21	22	23	24	25	26	27	28	29	30	35	40
	Weight (in pounds)													
Height	HEALTHY WEIGHT						OVERWEIGHT					OBESE		
4'10"	91	96	100	105	110	115	119	124	129	134	138	143	167	191
4'11"	94	99	104	109	114	119	124	128	133	138	143	148	173	198
5'0"	97	102	107	112	118	123	128	133	138	143	148	153	179	204
5'1"	100	106	111	116	122	127	132	137	143	148	153	158	185	211
5'2"	104	109	115	120	126	131	136	142	147	153	158	164	191	218
5'3"	107	113	118	124	130	135	141	146	152	158	163	169	197	225
5'4"	110	116	122	128	134	140	145	151	157	163	169	174	204	232
5'5"	114	120	126	132	138	144	150	156	162	168	174	180	210	240
5'6"	118	124	130	136	142	148	155	161	167	173	179	186	216	247
5'7"	121	127	134	140	146	153	159	166	172	178	185	191	223	255
5'8"	125	131	138	144	151	158	164	171	177	184	190	197	230	262
5'9"	128	135	142	149	155	162	169	179	182	189	196	203	236	270
5'10"	132	139	146	153	160	167	174	181	188	195	202	207	243	278
5'11"	136	143	150	157	165	172	179	186	193	200	208	215	250	286
6'0"	140	147	154	162	169	177	184	191	199	206	213	221	258	294
6'1"	144	151	159	166	174	182	189	197	204	212	219	227	265	302
6'2"	148	155	163	171	179	186	194	202	210	218	225	233	272	311
6'3"	152	160	168	176	184	192	200	208	216	224	232	240	279	319
6'4"	156	164	172	180	189	197	205	213	221	230	238	246	287	328
	Small Frame													
			Medium Frame											
				Large Frame										

Note: Height is measured without shoes and Weight is measured without clothes.

1. Dietary Guidelines Advisory Committee, 2000 Report and National Institutes of Health, 1998. The BMI (weight-for-height) ranges shown above are for adults. They are not exact ranges of healthy and unhealthy weights. However, they show that health risk increases at higher levels of overweight and obesity. Even within the healthy BMI range, weight gains can carry health risks for adults. Weight-for-frame-size is based on Metropolitan Life Insurance guidelines.

Table 3
BMI Table with Frame Sizes

Calories Count

Now that you've determined your goal weight, the next step is to find out how many calories you should be eating each day to reach that goal. Exercise or increased physical activity is going to be one of the components included in that number, and you'll see what a difference it can make.

Step 1: How many calories are you presently eating?

The first thing to do is determine how active you are. Read each of the following descriptions and see which one sounds most like you.

> Do you sit or stand around for long periods of time? Do you do some minimal physical activity about once a week? If so, you're a *sedentary* person.
>
> If you tend to be up and about most of the time, whether at home or on the job, and are involved in some form of exercise for at least 30 minutes a day, 2 to 3 times a week, you're a person who does *light* activity.

If your job requires a good deal of energy, and you like being active in your leisure time for at least 60 minutes a day, 3 to 5 times a week, you're a person who does *moderate* activity.

If your job involves manual labor, and you still enjoy being active during your leisure time for at least 60 minutes a day, 5 to 6 times a week, you're an *active* person.

As you go through the process of determining the number of calories you're presently eating, be sure that you assess your activity level correctly. Assessing your lifestyle as being more active than it is will mean that you're going to calculate your calorie requirements too high. Instead of losing weight, you could end up gaining. Find your activity level in the following table, making sure you look in the correct column for your gender.

Level of Activity	Women	Men
Sedentary	12	14
Light	13	15
Moderate	14	16
Active	15	17

Table 4
Multiplier for Calculating Calories

Multiply your present weight by the multiplier you found in Table 3. The result is the number of calories you're presently eating per day, i.e., a calorie level that's maintaining your present weight. Go ahead and fill in the blanks.

___________	X	___________	=	___________
Your Present Weight (pounds)		Multiplier		Daily Calories Being Eaten

For example, David weighs 205 pounds and does "light" activity. So, he multiplies 205 pounds by "15" (his multiplier), and finds out that, on average, he's eating about 3,075 calories per day to maintain his present weight.

205	X	15	=	3075
David's Weight (pounds)		Multiplier		Daily Calories Being Eaten by David

Step 2: How many calories should you be eating per day to lose weight?

Obviously, if you want to lose weight you have to eat fewer calories than you're presently eating. Subtract 500 calories from the number of calories you just calculated above. In David's case, he'd subtract 500 from 3,075 calories to find out that about 2,500 calories per day would be right for him to lose 1 pound per week. Now you do the calculations for you own daily required calorie level to lose weight:

___________	-	500 calories	=	___________
Your Present Calorie Requirement				Calories To Be Eaten Per Day to Lose Weight

You may be thinking, "It'll take me forever to lose the weight doing it as slowly as one pound per week." What you may not have considered is that when you add an exercise component to this plan—one where you burn about 200 to 300 calories per exercise session, and you exercise 5 days a week—you could lose up to about 1½ to 2 pounds per week, which is just right.

One important point to keep in mind when you're doing your calorie calculations: Women shouldn't eat fewer than 1,200 calories per day, no matter what the calculations come up with. And men shouldn't eat fewer than 1,500 calories per day. If the calorie intake goes too low, you won't get enough nutrition to keep your body healthy.

Setting Up The Daily Connection

You now know how many calories you should be eating per day. You also should have decided which diet you want to follow: *Low-Carb, Balanced,* or *Low-Fat.* What you do need to decide is at what percentage level you want carbohydrates or fat to be. My suggestion is to start out somewhere in the middle of each range. Since you can easily move your starting line, it's really up to you how drastic a change from what you're doing right now you want.

You'll be using this table to determine where to place your horizontal and vertical lines on *The Daily Connection:*

Calorie Level →		1200	1300	1400	1500	1600	1700	1800	1900	2000	2100	2200	2300	2400
Horizontal Line at:		24	26	28	30	32	34	36	38	40	42	44	46	48
DIET TYPE ↓		Vertical line at:												
Low-Carb Monitor Carbs	50%	18	19	21	22	24	25	27	28	30	31	33	34	36
	45%	16	17	19	20	21	23	24	25	27	28	29	31	32
	40%	14	15	17	18	19	20	21	23	24	25	26	27	29
	35%	13	14	15	16	17	18	19	20	21	22	23	24	25
Balanced Monitor Fat	35%	18	20	21	23	24	26	27	29	30	32	33	35	36
	30%	15	17	18	19	21	22	23	24	26	27	28	30	31
	25%	13	14	15	16	17	18	19	20	21	23	24	25	26
Low-Fat Monitor Fat	25%	13	14	15	16	17	18	19	20	21	23	24	25	26
	20%	10	11	12	13	14	15	15	16	17	18	19	20	21
	15%	8	8	9	10	10	11	12	12	13	14	14	15	15
	10%	5	6	6	6	7	7	8	8	9	9	9	10	10

Table 5
Numbers for Setting Up Your Daily Connection

Print a blank *Daily Connection (*you'll find the template in the Appendix) and do the following two steps:

1. Set Up for Calories

In the top row of Table 4 (see above), find the Calorie Level you should be having each day (the number you just calculated to lose weight). The row below that number says "Horizontal Line at:". What number does it show for your calorie level? Find that number on the **right-hand side** of *The Daily Connection* and circle it. Now draw a horizontal line all the way across *The Daily Connection*. Let's look at Riley's *Daily Connection* again. She is eating 1200 calories. From Table 4, she finds out she should circle "24" on the right-hand side. This is how her *Daily Connection* would look so far:

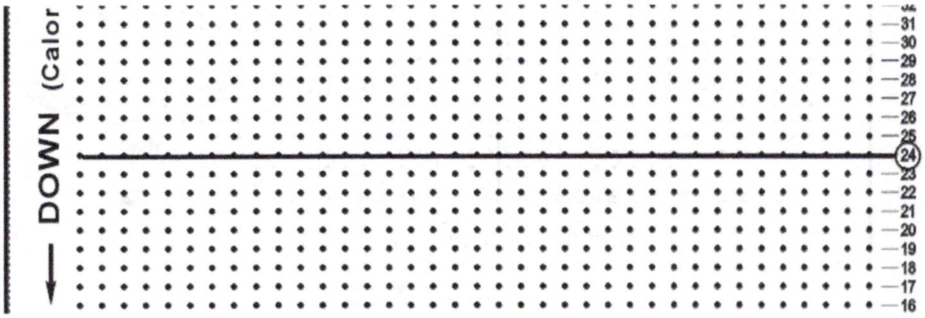

Figure 7
Setting Up for Calories

2. Set up for Carbohydrates or Fat

You should have decided by now whether you want to follow the *Low-Carb*, *Low-Fat* or *Balanced* diet.

Following a Low-Carb Diet

How strict a low-carb diet do you want to be on? As you can see from the Table 4 above, you can have a diet ranging from 35% to 50% of calories coming from carbohydrates. Consider starting at 45% to see how that works for you. If you find you're hungry all the time, decrease the percentage of carbs and increase the amount of protein you're eating.

For this step, again find the number of calories you should be eating per day at the top of the table. Follow that column down to the level of carbs you want to be eating. What number did you come to? That's the number to circle on the bottom part of *The Daily Connection*, the ACROSS numbers. Now draw a vertical line to the left of that number, between it and the next higher number. The reason for this is so you don't hide the dots you'll need for *drawing the line.*

As an example and mentioned earlier, Riley decided that she wants to follow the *Low-Carb* diet at the 50% level. Looking at Table 4, she finds that she needs to circle "18" at the bottom of *The Daily Connection* where you see the word "ACROSS".

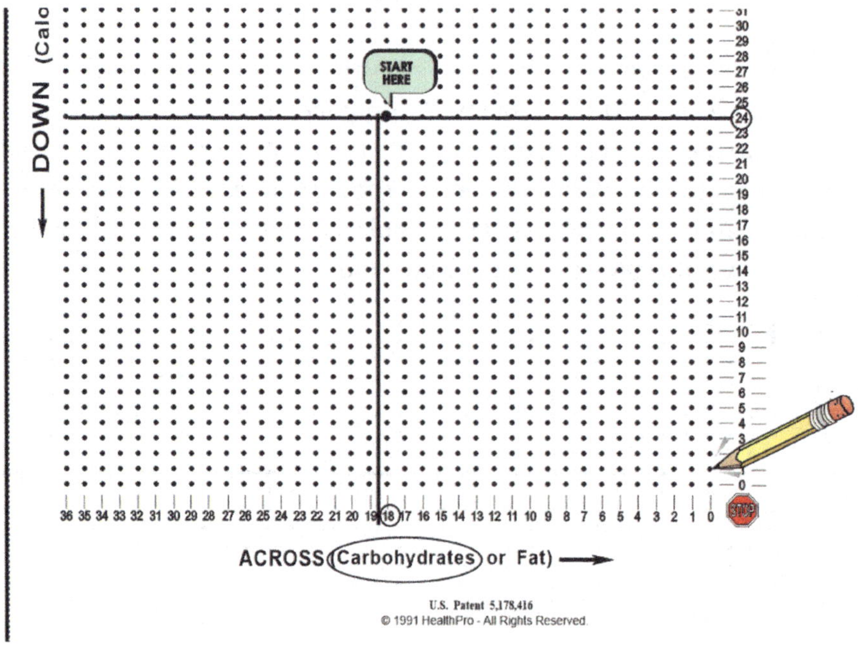

Figure 8
Setting Up for Carbohydrates (or Fat)

You might want to put the words "Start Here" when you embark on your *drawing the line* journey. Makes for a good visual.

If Riley finds that she gets hungry easily with a 50% carbohydrate diet, she can drop it down to 45% or less.

Following a Low-Fat or Balanced Diet

Both the *Low-Fat* and *Balanced* Diets monitor for fat. The difference between the two is based on how strict you want to be on your fat intake. For the *Low-Fat* diet, you can choose 10% to 25% of calories from fat. On the *Balanced* Diet, you can choose 25% to 35% of calories from fat. As with the *Low-Carb* diet, find the number of calories you should be eating per day at the top of the table. Follow that column down to the level of fat you want to be eating based on the diet approach you selected. Circle that number at the bottom of *The Daily Connection*; then draw a vertical line. The intersection of the two lines you've drawn is your **"Start Here"** point.

3. Label *The Daily Connection*

Don't forget to circle at the top of the page and at the bottom either "Carbohydrates" or "Fat" depending upon which diet you're following. By saving copies of *The Daily Connections* you create, you can visually see what has been working for you and what has not. I often eat the same breakfast every day. By doing that, I can just copy what I did for yesterday's breakfast without having to look the foods up in the Food List again.

Include the "Date", "Calories", and what % level of Carbohydrates or Fat you're intending to eat.

CHAPTER 3

Making the Most of *Drawing the Line*

Some Clever Tips

To get the most out of *The Daily Connection*, there are some things you can do that don't take much time but can have long-term value.

Include the name of the food on *The Daily Connection*

As you draw lines and circles to mark off the number of calories and carbs/fat you've eaten, it would be very helpful for you to write in the space to the left or right of the line what food you actually ate. It's a great way to record meal information. It's especially helpful if you repeat a meal. You won't need to look up the foods again. Just copy the DOWN and ACROSS lines from another *Daily Connection.* If you eat exactly the same foods on one day as you did on another, you don't need to make a chart for it. You already know that it works for you.

How often to *draw the line*

The idea with *Drawing the Line* is to show you what food choices work with your day's allowances for calories, carbs, and fat. I recommend you *draw the line* every day for at least 3 to 4 weeks. I'm sure your food choices will vary over that time and get you familiar with how your choices fit onto *The Daily Connection*. After you've got a feel for this, then consider *drawing the line* twice a week (one weekday and one weekend day). Either continue to do it once a week or quit and only consider revisiting the process if you're not reaching your goals or find yourself backsliding. Of course, if you set a new goal, then I'd go back to doing it every day to get used to what that new approach looks and feels like.

Using different colored pencils

Consider using different colored pens or pencils when you draw the circles. Use one color for breakfast, another for your snack, another for lunch, and so on. It's a great way of tracking what portion of your calories you eat at what times of the day. If you want to be more proactive, do actual meal planning for the whole day.

Meal Planning for Calories

The idea with any effective weight-loss plan is to lose weight in a way that doesn't make you hungry all the time. Even though signs of hunger are good, since it tells you it's time to eat, being hungry all the time means you're not eating enough calories to match the calories you're burning. Consider dividing up your calorie intake for the day, either distributing those calories more evenly throughout the day or in a way that accounts for when you know you'll need the calories the most. It's really up to you how you want to divide up your calories.

An easy way to give this a try is simply divide your daily calorie allowance (the number of calorie "dots" you've drawn the horizontal line for) by 3. Now you have breakfast, lunch, and dinner allocated for. If you decide you need to have a snack in the morning or the afternoon, "steal" a couple of dots from your next meal.

Look at the following *Daily Connection* that shows an example of someone who has drawn horizontal lines for 3 meals and 2 snacks for the day, dividing up the calories accordingly. If the foods are selected wisely, when the last circle is drawn for the food in a meal or a snack, it won't go over the horizontal line for that meal or snack.

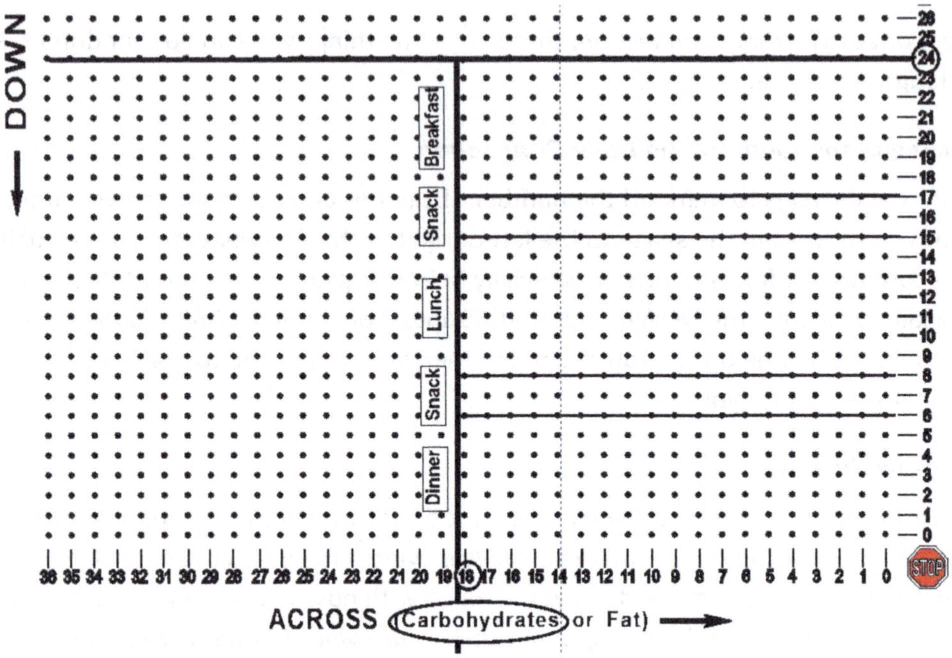

Figure 9
An Example of Meal Planning According to Calories

Meal Planning for Carbohydrates

If you're someone who has diabetes or has been diagnosed as pre-diabetic, possibly with insulin resistance, you've probably been told that you need to keep your carbohydrate intake under strict control. Since carbs become glucose in the bloodstream, counting and limiting the amount of carbs you eat at any one time can help avoid too much of a rise in your blood glucose. *Drawing the Line* makes counting carbs easy to do. But even for someone who doesn't have diabetes, spacing your carbohydrates out throughout the day will give you a more uniform level of energy.

Your choice of carbohydrates will also make a difference. There are two types of carbohydrates — simple and complex. Sugar is an example of a simple carbohydrate. Legumes, beans, whole grain foods are examples of complex carbohydrates. Simple carbohydrates are quickly digested and metabolized, leading to spikes in blood sugar. Complex carbohydrates take longer to be digested and metabolized and therefore help blood sugar stay at a more even level.

So, no matter whether you have diabetes or not, it is helpful to divide your day up according to carbohydrates (just as you did with calories).

Meal Planning for Carb Counting

The term, "meal planning," is the same thing as saying "carb counting," since you are planning ahead for how many carbs you will be eating at any particular time. You divide up *The Daily Connection* with "carbohydrate lines" (which are vertical lines). You just learned how to draw "calorie lines" or horizontal lines — Figure 8. This is an easy way to achieve your goal of controlling your blood glucose.

You need to determine how many grams of carbohydrates you should have for each meal or snack. If you have diabetes, you may want to work with your healthcare provider or dietitian since he or she will know what medications you're on in order to match it correctly with your food intake. Once you know how many grams you should have for the various meals and snacks, check out Table 5, which shows how those grams of carbohydrates translate into dots. Each dot covers a certain range of carb grams.

Grams of carbs per meal			Count over this many dots, then draw a vertical line
1	to	4	0
5	to	12	1
13	to	20	2
21	to	29	3
30	to	37	4
38	to	46	5
47	to	54	6
55	to	62	7
63	to	71	8
72	to	75	9

Table 6
Carb Counting on The Daily Connection

Let's watch what Steve does. He was advised by his dietitian that he should be eating 1800 calories with 40% of those calories coming from carbohydrates. That 40% carbohydrates is equivalent to 180 grams of carbohydrates that need to be distributed in a sensible way throughout the day. The dietitian suggested the following:

- Breakfast: 48 grams
- Snack: 20 grams
- Lunch: 46 grams
- Dinner: 46 grams
- Snack: 21 grams

Steve's next step is to mark off on *The Daily Connection* how those grams of carbohydrates translate into dots. Referring to Table 5, we now take the recommendation of Steve's dietitian and convert those grams into dots.

- Breakfast: 48 grams = 6 dots
- Snack: 20 grams = 2 dots
- Lunch: 46 grams = 5 dots
- Dinner: 46 grams = 5 dots
- Snack: 20 grams = 3 dots

Look at Figure 9 to see how Steve drew the vertical lines to delineate how many ACROSS dots (carbohydrates) he gets for each meal.

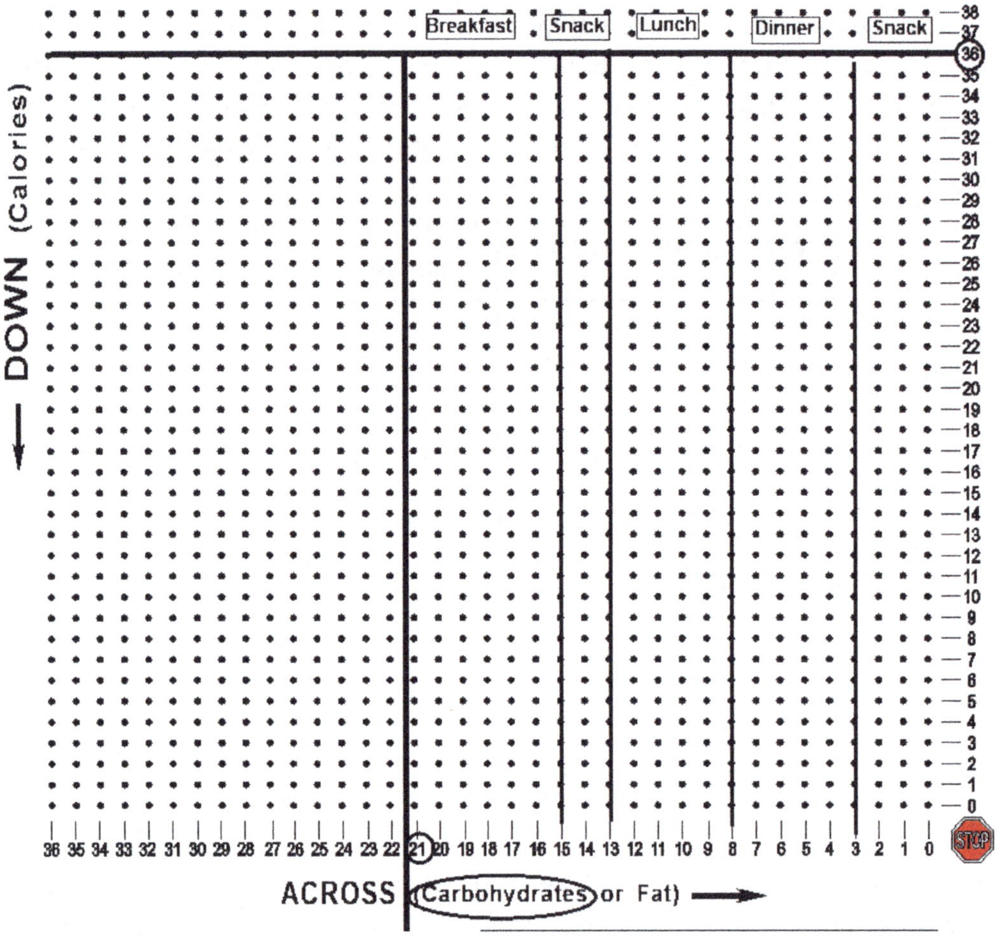

Figure 10

An Example of Meal Planning with Carb Counting (1800 calories / 40% Carbohydrates)

Of course, your *Daily Colleciton* may look different depending upon your calorie intake and percentage carbohydrates you've chosen. As with meal planning for calories, your last circle for a particular meal or snack should not go over the vertical line allowed for that eating period. This is when the *Food List* sorted from "Least to Most Carbohydrates" will be most helpful.

Monitoring Your Blood Glucose

Knowing how much carbohydrate you're eating is just one piece of the puzzle. If you have diabetes or even pre-diabetes, monitoring your blood glucose is another very important piece of that puzzle. It's generally accepted that a fasting or pre-meal plasma blood glucose value should be somewhere between 90 and 130 mg/dl. A post-meal plasma blood glucose level, taken 1-2 hours after the start of the meal, should be less than 180 mg/dl. Ask your healthcare provider to help you set fasting, pre-meal and post meal blood glucose level goals.

The Daily Connection includes a place for people with diabetes to keep track of their blood glucose levels throughout the day as you can see in Figure 10. The vertical lines are those drawn after each meal as you saw Steve do in Figure 9.

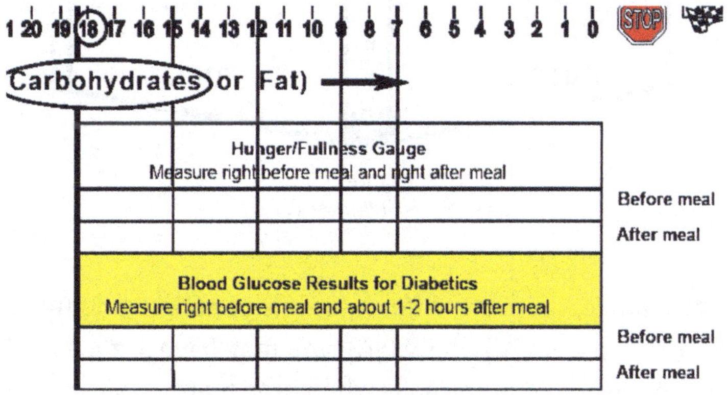

Figure 11
Tracking Blood Glucose for Each Meal

If you have diabetes, take *The Daily Connection* with you to your healthcare professional or dietitian so they can see what foods you're eating and the resulting blood glucose. This one page of information tells so much about how your body is dealing with glucose and how you might need to make adjustments. Maybe going on a lower-carb diet or possibly a high-fat diet would help.

Gauging Your Hunger and Fullness

You might have noticed the "Hunger-Fullness" Gauge on *The Daily Connection.* This is another bit of tracking you can do, helping you to become more mindful of when you're hungry enough to eat. Are you really hungry when you started eating? Were you overly full when you finished eating?

I created this gauge in a way that "Satisfied" or pretty close to Satisfied is where you should start eating and stop eating. Starting to eat when you're "Very Hungry (VH)" or even "Starving (St)" is bound to get you into trouble. You've waited too long to eat and you'll probably gobble down whatever it is you decided to eat. And with that, you won't be able to recognize when you've just reached the "Satisfied (S)" level. It takes at least 20 minutes for any food that went through the stomach and arrived in the intestine to send messages to the brain that food is on its way. Think of how much food you could eat in 20 minutes. Probably far more than your body really needs to get your blood sugar up to normal. There's a tip right there — eat slowly to give your body time to react to the arriving food and send the necessary messages.

By the way, recognizing fullness is just as crucial as being aware of when you're hungry. It's probably even more so, since ignoring fullness signals leads to eating excess calories. The next time you eat, refer to the following Hunger-Fullness Gauge to find out where your hunger needle is pointing.

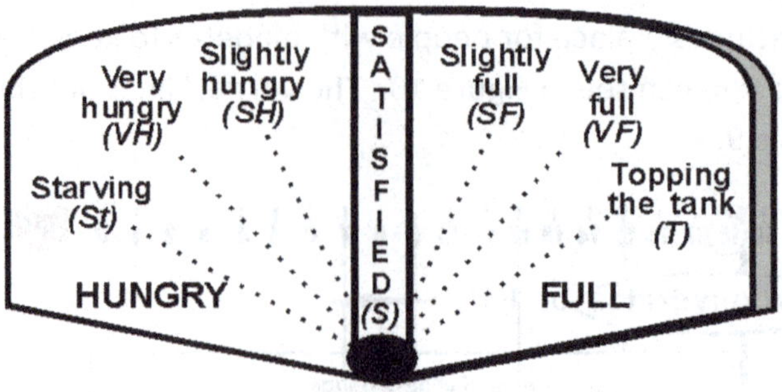

Figure 12
Hunger-Fullness Gauge

As you can see from the gauge, there are different levels of hunger and fullness and the feelings that go with those levels. When you're Slightly hungry (SH), you may have a somewhat empty feeling, but not much more than that. Very hungry (VH) is normally when others are also aware of your needing food—your stomach is growling and grumbling. If you're at the Starving (St) stage, you may be dizzy or feeling faint.

On the other side of the gauge are the relative levels of fullness. When you're Slightly full (SF), there's a somewhat heavy feeling in your stomach and awareness that hunger has already been taken care of many bites ago. Very full (VF) is where you're starting to get uncomfortable, having a sensation of a very-stretched stomach. By the time you reach Topping the tank (T), you've really overdone it. It's the same feeling you have on Thanksgiving, when you feel you just can't budge, where breathing is a little harder and you definitely are feeling gastric distress.

Notice that right in the middle of the two sides of the gauge is an area called "Satisfied (S)". At this spot on the gauge, you're neither hungry nor full. You're feeling just right. That's the target range you're shooting for. Keep that in mind as you eat.

There is a problem with starting to eat when you're in the *Satisfied* range. You inevitably end up on the *Full* side of the gauge. The way this gauge is created, and the way you should think about eating, is that you should never end up in the Full range. Satisfied is as far as you should go. By eating into the Full range, you're consuming more food than your body needs. Remember, *Satisfied* is where you should be!

So at what point should you start eating? Eating when you get to *Slightly hungry* is the best place, since you probably won't need to eat much to arrive back at *Satisfied*.

If you wait until *Very hungry* or *Starving*, you're asking for trouble. Your choice of foods might not be as healthy. You might eat the first thing you see, even if it's not the best for you. Why do you think fast food restaurants do so well? They cater to those who need food quickly, no matter whether it's the best choice or not.

Logging Hunger and Fullness

Just as there is a place to log in your blood glucose (if you're measuring it), there is also a place to log in your level of hunger and fullness. By drawing a line down through the dots and the Hunger/Fullness table, you can keep track on *The Daily Connection* of your hunger and fullness before and after the meal or snack. It becomes a wake-up call when you realize that you're eating when you're not hungry.

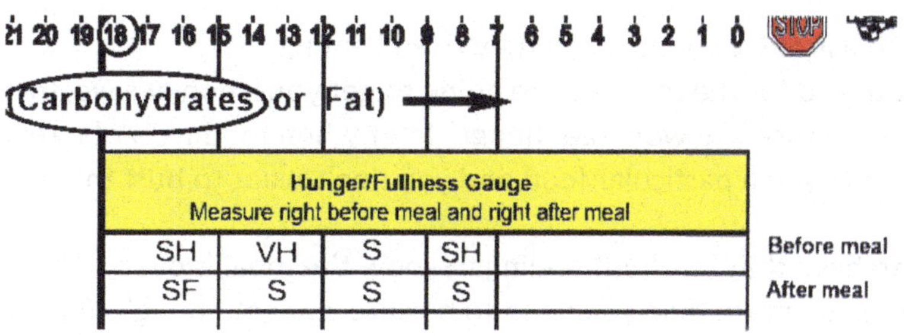

Figure 13
An Example of Meal Planning with Carb Counting (1800 calories / 40% Carbohydrates)

Recognizing the "Satisfied" Level

What will it take for you to realize that you're at the *Satisfied* level once you've started eating? If there's no true bodily sensation as you'd have with being really full (stomach stretched, feeling drowsy, uncomfortable), then how do you know when to stop? One of the first steps in this plan requires that you have your undivided attention on the eating process. There's no way you can recognize being *Satisfied* if your mind is elsewhere. Watching television or reading a book is too much of a distraction to keep you focused. Besides, if you went through the trouble of preparing something to eat, why not be mindful of it and focus on how you're enjoying it?

Next, you need to do what you can to slow down your eating process. It takes at least 20 minutes for the first bites of food to send signals to your brain that food is on its way. After each bite, try to sense whether you've reached the *Satisfied* level (contented but not heavy or stretched feeling). One very clever way to slow yourself down is to eat your meal with the opposite hand from the one you normally use. After dropping food in your lap once or twice because of trying to keep up with your usual pace, you'll have to slow down. You could also use a smaller fork or spoon, such as a cocktail fork or baby spoon. Try putting your fork down between bites and asking yourself the question, "Have I had enough yet?" Maybe even try chopsticks.

If You Aren't Hungry, Why Are You Eating?

The reasons people eat when they're not hungry are so numerous, that it would probably fill an entire book. Here are some of the more obvious reasons for why we start eating when not hungry or continue eating when we're full:

- A food's smell
- The sight of food
- Feeling you always have to have dessert even if you're full just to have a sweet taste in your mouth
- Being bored
- Eating to stay awake
- There's still food left on the plate
- Trying to satisfy thirst with food
- Using food as a transition activity—a way of avoiding starting something
- Using food to deal with emotional issues
- Fear of not getting a particular food again
- Using food as a reward for doing a good job
- Eating a particular food whenever a specific event occurs (for example, popcorn at the movies)

- Dining with a group of people and they're still eating
- Feeling you paid for the food, you're going to get your money's worth
- Wanting to be sure you won't get hungry later when food won't be readily available
- A friend made you a particular food and you don't want to hurt that person's feelings by not eating it
- Needing to have that "stuffed" feeling to know the meal is over
- Serving yourself more than you need to be sure you get enough (for example, serving "family style" or going out for Chinese food)
- Not wanting to waste food
- Not wanting to have leftovers
- Eating so quickly that your body doesn't recognize how much food it has had
- With various distractions (conversation, television, etc.), lack of awareness of how much is being eaten
- The food came in a "serving-sized" package
- Tasting food while you're cooking it
- Finding that the container you're storing the leftovers in isn't quite large enough, so you eat what doesn't fit
- You're programmed to eat by the clock
- Eating all foods on a prescribed weight-loss plan because you believe you have to

Any you'd like to add?

CHAPTER 4

Getting Physical

On its most basic level, losing weight is a matter of "*calories in* versus *calories out*." I do appreciate that there are many variables to consider with weight loss on the individual level. However, the concept of calories in/calories out gives you a good starting point. Your body needs so many calories of food just to run. It's often referred to as your "resting metabolism". Even when you're just lying in bed, your heart is still pumping, your lungs are still breathing, and a host of many other functions are working even though we're never aware of them.

Now let's throw physical activity into the mix. Depending upon what you choose to do, from a simple stroll in the park to mountain climbing, you're going to need extra calories to accomplish it. In Chapter 2 you found out what your total calories should be based on the level of your activity (sedentary, light, moderate, or active). Now you have a chance to get a bit more specific about your activity and its effect on the calories you're burning.

Physical activity or regular exercise in whatever form that increases your heart rate is good for you (unless you've been told otherwise by your doctor). It doesn't hurt to check with your physician before embarking on an exercise program. What you do for exercise can be anything you enjoy doing and will stick with. The last point is the important one. You have to enjoy something to continue to do it. Also, it doesn't have to be the same activity every day. In fact, it's better if you vary the activity and let all the different muscles have a bit of exercise. One day, focus on doing aerobics, such as jogging or biking — getting your heart rate somewhere in the range of 70-80% of your maximum heart rate.

> To calculate your Maximum Heart Rate: Subtract your age from 220. Then multiply by 70% up to 80% to find a comfortable, but aerobic, exercise heart rate. Either check your pulse on your wrist or at the carotid artery on your neck to confirm you're achieving that rate.

On another day, work on weight-lifting — helping to build up your body mass. Follow an exercise session with stretching and flexibility exercises to stay limber. A good weekly routine would be to do aerobics on Mondays, Wednesdays, and Fridays for at least 30 minutes. Follow that with maybe 10-15 minutes of flexibility exercises. Then, on Tuesdays and Thursdays, do weight-lifting or resistance training with about 15-20 minutes of aerobics. On the weekend, do something new. Rock-climbing anyone?

Exercise is good for everyone but especially for someone with diabetes, because even if you're on diabetes medications, exercise helps move glucose out of the bloodstream and into the cells. Some people with diabetes who exercise can often lower the amount of medication they take. Exercise will often help people with heart disease or high blood pressure decease their medication, as well.

Drawing the Line will help you track your exercise in a similar way that you track your food except it's done in the opposite direction (see Figure 13 on the next page.) Instead of *drawing the line* DOWN on the sheet, this time you'll be *drawing the line* UP. I'm not setting any limits on how much you want to exercise. As you look at *The Daily Connection,* notice the numbers on the left. That shows the amount of food calories that are getting burned off with the the exercise. Each dot is worth 50 calories.

Hopefully this approach will encourage you to exercise more since the more you exercise, the more calories you burn!

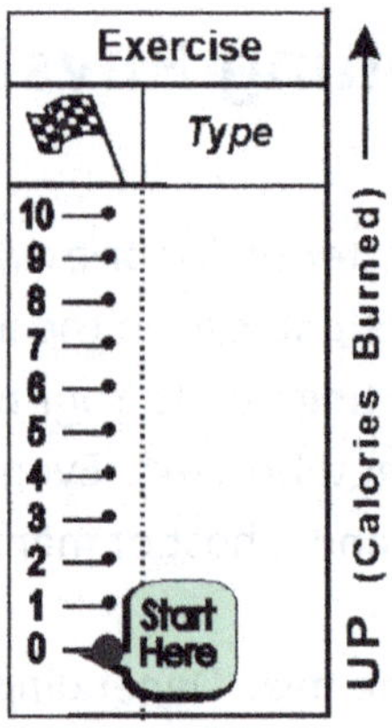

Figure 14
Tracking Your Exercise

Tracking Your Exercise

Because exercise burns calories, in order to track it on your *Daily Connection*, you need to know how to calculate the dots of exercise you do. The number of dots will be based on the type of exercise and how much you weigh. The heavier you are, the more calories you'll burn doing the same exercise as someone who weighs less than you. You'll be using the information in Table 6 — "Multipliers for Calculating Dots of Exercise" — following these three steps:

Step 1: Locate the exercise you want to do in Table 6. Then run your finger across to the number in the column titled, "Calories Burned per Pound per Minute." Multiply that number by your weight (in pounds) to find out how many calories you burned *per minute* for that particular exercise.

Step 2: Multiply the result you just got in Step 1 by the number of minutes you exercised to determine the total number of calories burned in that length of time.

Step 3: Divide the result you got in Step 2 by 50. This gives you how many dots of exercise you did, a number you will use to track your exercise on *The Daily Connection*.

Activity	Calories Burned Per Pound Per Minute	Activity	Calories Burned Per Pound Per Minute
Badminton	0.04	Scrubbing floors	0.05
Bicycling, 10 mph	0.05	Scuba diving	0.06
Chopping wood, ax	0.04	Skating, ice	0.04
Dancing, ballroom	0.03	Skiing, cross-country	0.06
Dancing, modern	0.04	Skiing, downhill	0.04
Gardening, hoe, dig	0.05	Snow shoveling, light	0.05
Golf, walking	0.04	Snowshoe walking	0.08
Hiking, hilly	0.06	Soccer	0.06
Horse grooming	0.06	Squash	0.07
Horseback riding, trot	0.05	Swimming, slow crawl	0.06
House cleaning	0.03	Table tennis	0.03
Jogging, 6 mph	0.07	Tennis, doubles	0.03
Jumping rope	0.06	Tennis, singles	0.05
Mopping	0.03	Volleyball	0.04
Painting, outside	0.04	Walking, 3.5 mph	0.04
Racquetball	0.07	Waterskiing	0.05
Rowing machine	0.05	Weight training	0.03
Sawing, by hand	0.06		

Table 7
Multipliers for Calculating Dots of Exercise

Let's go through the example of Tami, who decided to take a brisk walk for an hour. In Table 6 she found that "Walking, 3.5 mph" burns *0.04 calories per minute per pound*. Tami weighs 155 pounds. The following is what she did to determine the number of dots she would track on her *Daily Connection*:

Step 1: 0.04 x 155 pounds = 6.2 calories per minute

Step 2: 6.2 x 60 minutes = 372 calories

Step 3: 372 calories / 50 calories per dot = 7.4 dots
(Tami rounds this to 7 dots for tracking purposes. Had it been 7.5 to 7.9, she'd round up to 8 dots)

Remember that if you're on medication, it's important to talk with your healthcare provider to determine whether you will need to adjust your medication because of the increased exercise.

CHAPTER 5

Becoming Food Savvy

Most people rarely think about what is in the food they're eating. Nor do they consider what nutritional value their food choices have on their health. Most of us grew up learning in school about the various food groups. The government tries with its *Dietary Guidelines for Americans* to give Americans an idea of what a healthy diet would include. The USDA (United States Department of Agriculture) shares on its website at www.myplate.gov healthy ways to eat. I highly recommend you check it out. Do you remember the Food Guide Pyramid? It's now been replaced with MyPlate, the official symbol of the five food groups.

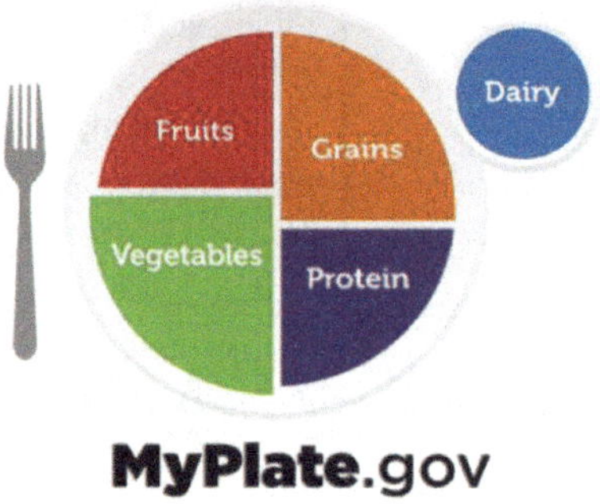

How Sweet It Is

When you visit the government website, you can click on each food group to see healthy suggestions. For now, I want to discuss sugar because it seems to get included in one form or another in almost all processed foods. It's one thing to get sugar from fruit. It's naturally occurring and along with that sugar (mostly in the form of *fructose)* you get a lot of vitamins and minerals and fiber. The same cannot be said about the sugar found in sweetened cereals, for example. The following is a list, which I like to call "Sugar by Another Name is Still Sugar":

- Beet sugar
- Brown sugar
- Cane sugar
- Concentrated fruit juice
- Confectioner's sugar
- Crystallized cane juice
- Dextrin
- Dextrose
- Evaporated cane juice
- Fructose
- High fructose corn syrup
- Honey
- Invert sugar
- Levulose
- Maltodextrin

- Maple syrup
- Molasses
- Raw sugar
- Sucrose
- Table sugar
- Turbinado sugar
- White sugar

Sugar-Free Foods

Having diabetes doesn't mean you have to eat only sugar-free foods. Yet, keep in mind the common misconception of many dieters — that all sugar-free foods are carbohydrate-free or even calorie-free. They aren't. There are many *no-calorie sweeteners* that are part of the line-up of ingredients in sugar-free foods: acesulfame-potassium, aspartame, neotame, saccharin, and sucralose. Recent research is showing that these sugar substitutes actually cause people to become hungrier. That's because the food may taste sweet, but the brain has not been fooled. It was looking for calories when it stimulated the hunger growls and it has not been satisfied.

Researchers are also finding that the gut bacteria aren't too pleased with sugar substitutes. They can possibly cause a condition called "leaky gut" where certain molecules get past the intestinal wall, molecules that shouldn't.

Better to train your taste buds to less sugar. Believe it or not, the body can be very adaptable. People who have cut down on the amount of fat they eat find that fried foods just taste too greasy for them now.

The Myth of Fat Phobia

Even though *Drawing the Line* is a system about controlling for calories, carbs and fat, it's also about eating healthfully. Too much fat and the wrong kinds of fat can potentially be harmful to your health. Back in the 1970s, the public was advised to cut fat out of the diet because it was considered bad for us. It was thought that it fostered an increase in cholesterol and made us physically fat. So, food manufacturers were only too happy to provide us with low-fat and no-fat foods. But when they cut out the fat, they added sugar for flavor. Sometimes a low-fat food didn't have fewer calories than its regular fat version, but it could boast about its low-fat content.

While certain fats are bad for people, such as saturated and trans fats, there are some that are essential to a normal diet. One benefit of having healthy fats in the diet is that they help transport through the body the necessary fat-soluble nutrients like vitamins A, D, E and K, as well as beta-carotene. Moreover, many of us enjoy eating fats because they give food some of its flavor. They also help with satiety (a feeling of fullness).

Saturated fats are found in abundance in meats, high-fat dairy products (e.g., cheeses, ice cream and butter) and in some tropical oils (coconut oil, palm oil and palm kernel oil). One way to recognize saturated fats is that they're solid at room temperature. Eating too much of these can increase your risk for heart disease, because they can potentially elevate total blood cholesterol. Saturated fats tend to increase the "bad" LDL-cholesterol in your blood, a type of cholesterol that clogs your arteries. At the same time, they decrease the "good" HDL-cholesterol, the type that is necessary to remove the bad cholesterol from your blood. This is definitely not a good combination.

Monounsaturated fats are found in olive, canola, peanut and other nut oils. They tend to lower Total Cholesterol and LDL-cholesterol when the rest of your diet is low in saturated fats and calories. Obviously, this is beneficial.

Polyunsaturated fats consist of the omega-3 and omega-6 fatty acids. The omega-3s are found in ground flax seed, walnuts, cold-water fatty fish such as salmon, tuna, sardines, halibut, and herring, and in various oils (flax seed, soybean, canola and walnut). These fats help lower your risk of heart disease by decreasing the stickiness of blood platelets (decreasing your risk of blood clots), as well as by lowering triglycerides. The omega-6 fatty acids found in liquid corn, safflower, and soybean oils help lower total cholesterol, as well as LDL-cholesterol. Unfortunately, they also lower the good HDL-cholesterol, which means you should try to eat more of the omega-3s when possible.

Trans fatty acids (or ***trans fats***) had gotten a lot of attention in the past. They act like saturated fats, increasing the bad LDL-cholesterol and lowering the good HDL-cholesterol. They're even worse than saturated fat. Thankfully, the government has now restricted food manufacturers from adding trans fats to foods. From a food manufacturer's point-of-view, adding trans fat made oils more solid at room temperature. They also helped foods be more shelf-stable. Now that they have been restricted, manufacturers have to configure their foods differently. Let's face it. When you eat foods that are closer to how they came out of the ground, you're the better for it.

A discussion of fat would not be complete without mentioning **dietary cholesterol**. There is no good or bad cholesterol in food. It only becomes good (HDL-cholesterol) or bad (LDL-cholesterol) in your body. The only foods in which you'll find dietary cholesterol are animal products (meat, poultry, dairy products, seafood and eggs). Studies have shown that dietary cholesterol causes less of an increase in blood cholesterol than saturated fats do. That's why it's so important to watch how much saturated fat you're getting in your diet. Many people avoid shellfish because it's fairly high in cholesterol; yet, it's low in saturated fats. So there's no reason you can't enjoy shellfish unless you're allergic to it.

Healthy Food Choices

You now know what your calorie allowance is for the day (having calculated it in Chapter 2). The question is—How are you going to spend those calories? You could just as easily spend them on junk food as you could on healthy food choices. But obviously the junk food isn't going to give you the balanced nutrition you need.

Selecting healthy foods is as easy as 1-2-3-4-5. Every day, try to have at least:

1. **1** serving of dry beans (½ cup cooked)
2. **2** servings of low-fat or skim dairy product (e.g., 1 cup milk, 1 cup yogurt, 1½ ounces cheese)
3. **3** servings of fruit (e.g., 1 medium fresh, ½ cup canned without syrup, ¼ cup dried, ¾ cup juice)
4. **4** servings of whole grain foods (e.g., 1 slice bread, 1 oz cereal, ½ cup cooked pasta or rice)
5. **5** servings of vegetables (1 cup raw, ½ cup cooked, ½ cup frozen, ¾ cup juice)

These numbers may vary slightly, depending upon your daily calorie allowance, but the 1-2-3-4-5 approach gives you a base from which to work. When selecting fats, choose monounsaturated and polyunsaturated fats over saturated and trans fats. Keep sugar intake to a minimum—basically because it's just empty calories.

There's a place on your *Daily Connection*, "Food Groups," to keep track of how many servings of each of these types of food you eat. While you can eat more of each group than there are boxes, at least you'll know you've eaten the suggested minimum number of servings by the end of the day.

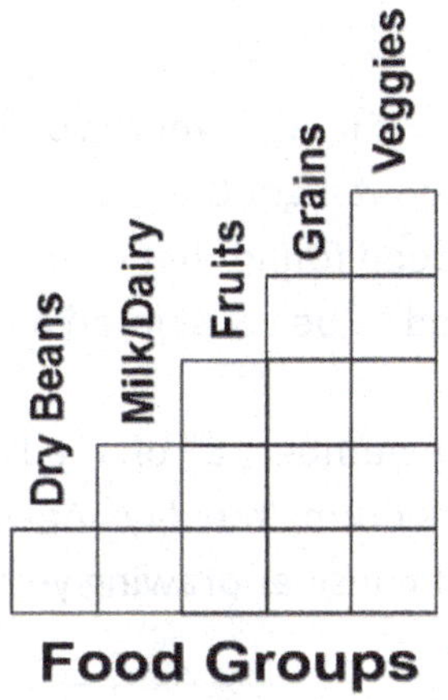

Figure 15
Tracking Food Groups on The Daily Connection

Having Your Protein

There is no mention of protein choices in the list above because most Americans get more than enough protein in their diet. There's protein in the dry beans, dairy foods, whole grains and even vegetables. Obviously, vegetarians do just fine without meat sources of protein. But, if you're a carnivore, enjoy your protein selections. Just try to make them low-fat versions since fat in meat is mostly saturated fat.

Beef: Eye of round, top round, tip roast, bottom round, top loin steak, arm roast, tenderloin, and flank steak *instead of* regular ground beef, brisket, untrimmed and highly-marbled cuts, ribs, sirloin, rib eye steak, London broil, blade roast, porterhouse steak, and T-bone steak.

Poultry: Go for breast without skin *instead of* legs, thighs and cuts with skin.

Pork: Try tenderloin, top loin roast, top loin chop, back loin ribs, and Canadian bacon or ham (that is, unless salt is a problem for you) *instead of* spareribs, shoulder blade steak, loin rib chop, sirloin roast, sausage, and bacon.

When it comes to **Fish**, the fattier the fish, the better a source of the omega-3 fatty acids it is. Try to include about 12 ounces of fish each week. Select such fish as catfish, pollock, salmon and light tuna, also shrimp more often since they have lower levels of mercury as compared to albacore tuna, swordfish or tilefish.

Choosing Your Food Groups for Meal Planning

One other suggestion is to consider your meals and snacks in terms of food choices: protein, starch, fruits and vegetables.

For breakfast, include a protein (e.g., egg, ham, turkey sandwich meat, cheese), a starch (e.g., toast, cereal, crackers), and a fruit (fresh, dried or canned).

For lunch, include a protein, starch, vegetable (e.g., raw carrots, broccoli, snap peas, string beans, cauliflower, or cooked vegetables), and fruit.

The same would go for dinner.

When having a snack, consider having a protein and a starch together rather than just a starch or fruit alone—the combination will control your blood sugar better. Also, include at least two dairy servings a day (e.g., milk, yogurt, cheese) as part of your meals or snacks.

Staying Hydrated

There's a place on *The Daily Connection* for "Fluids," where you can keep track of how much you drink each day. On average, you should drink about eight 8-ounce glasses of some beverage per day. That can include water, juice, coffee, tea, etc. It's been found that even caffeinated beverages can be considered part of your fluid intake for the day. It used to be considered a dehydrating liquid, but recently that thought has been disavowed.

To *draw the line* for fluids, start at the number "8" on the Daily Connection for "Fluids" and draw circles all the way down to "0" as you drink during the day. Again, this suggestion is a minimum. If you're eating more than 2000 calories, you might consider drawing your beginning line at the number "10."

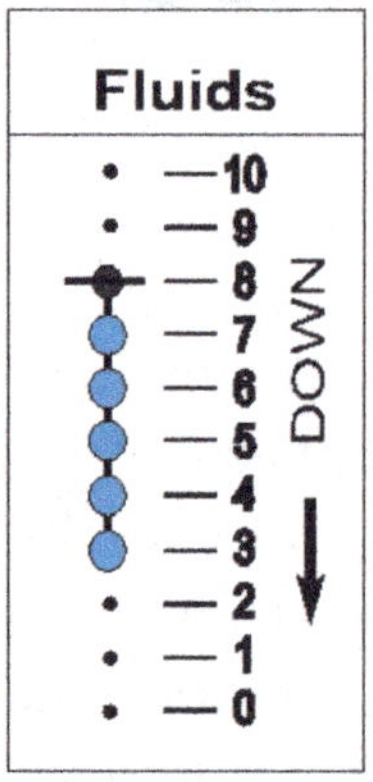

Figure 16

Tracking Fluids on The Daily Connection

Dining Out

Dining out might seem like a challenge, because how will you know how many calories you're eating? Here are some ideas. In fast food restaurants, you can ask for their Nutrition Facts brochure, which will provide you with calorie, total carbohydrate and total fat numbers. Then you can use the *Food Label Conversion Table* (Table 7) to convert the Nutrition Facts to dots to use on your *Daily Connection*.

If the restaurant doesn't offer nutrition information, look in the Food List in the Appendix to find a food that comes as close as possible to what you're planning on eating. It may not be the exact number of dots as the food you want to eat, but you're much better off *drawing the line* for something that's close than ignoring it altogether. Just remember—even if you don't track it, your body still knows you had it.

The following lists show different preparation styles that might appear on a menu. These lists can help you in making healthier choices. And if the information on the menu doesn't give you enough of an idea of how something is prepared, ask your waitperson. If you don't want something fried, find out if it can be grilled or baked. Another tip would be to ask for dressings, sauces and toppings to be served "on the side". Dip your fork into the dressing or sauce before you pick up the food. You'll end up eating much less of what you're dipping into, but the food will still taste just as great.

Have you ever stared at a menu, and only the appetizers sounded appealing? Then make a meal of just appetizers. Here's another planning idea: go online to the restaurant's website and check out the menu ahead of time. That will give you time to "study" the menu to determine what might be the best choices. On-the-spot ordering (when the restaurant smells so good and you're hungry) can often be troublesome.

Avoid These Methods of Preparation

- Alfredo sauce
- Au gratin
- Battered and fried
- Béchamel sauce
- Breaded and fried
- Butter sauce
- Buttered
- Buttery
- Casserole
- Cheese sauce
- Cream sauce
- Crème fraiche
- Crispy
- Deep-fried
- Escalloped
- Fried to a golden crust
- Fritters
- Guacamole sauce
- Hash
- Hollandaise sauce
- In drawn butter
- In pastry crust
- Made with butter
- Made with coconut milk
- Mayonnaise sauce
- Newburg
- Pan-fried
- Phyllo dough
- Pot pie
- Prime
- Sizzling
- Stuffed
- Stuffed and fried
- Stuffed with cheese
- Tempura style
- Thermidor
- Topped with shredded cheese
- With bacon or sausage
- With sour cream

- Wrapped in pastry dough

Try These Methods of Preparation Instead

- Au jus
- Baked
- Barbecued
- Blackened
- Boiled
- Braised
- Broiled
- Cajun style
- Charbroiled
- En brochette
- Fish sauce
- Grilled
- Hot sauce
- In clear broth
- In its own juices
- Kabobs or skewered
- Marinara sauce
- Marinated
- Poached
- Roasted
- Sautéed
- Served with salsa
- Simmered
- Smoked
- Steamed
- Stir-fried (ask chef to go easy on the oil)
- Vegetarian style
- With herbs

Drawing the Line on Recipes

Tracking foods included in a recipe can be done in the same DOWN-and-ACROSS approach on your *Daily Connection*. Take the amount of each ingredient and divide it by the number of servings per recipe. For example, if a recipe serves 4 people and calls for 1 cup of orange juice, then divide that one cup by 4 and *draw the line* for ¼ cup of orange juice (having checked for the number of dots in the Food List or on a food package label). Do the same thing for all the ingredients.

If you prefer, add up all the dots for calories for the complete recipe. Then divide by the number of servings to determine the number of dots to "draw the line" for. The same can be done for carbs and fat. It's up to you which way works best.

CHAPTER 6

Measuring Success — Rewarding Success

While you should see the results of your weight-loss efforts in how your clothes fit and how much more energy you'll have, it doesn't hurt to keep a weight-loss log. It gives some reality and numbers to what you're seeing. With that said, you really shouldn't weigh yourself more than once a week. Considering that losing about 2 pounds per week is about right, your scale isn't going to be sensitive enough for you to see, on average, 1/3 of a pound lost per day. Besides, there's no need to worship the scale, which is what the experience becomes when you do it every day. In fact, it can be emotionally defeating to weigh yourself too often. Many people determine what kind of day they're going to have based on the results of that morning weigh-in. Therefore, it's recommended you weigh yourself, at most, once a week, on the same day, preferably in the morning after you've gone to the bathroom and without clothes on.

A typical scale isn't that good a tool for measuring your progress anyway. The objective in weight loss is to get rid of the excess fat, as well as maintain and build muscle. The typical scale only measures your weight in pounds, without giving you any idea of how much of that weight is fat. Those pounds can be influenced by many things. There may be times when the scale tells you you're not losing any weight, no matter how good you've been following your diet plan. Yet, if you've been exercising, you're building muscle, which is heavier than fat. It could be that on a particular day you're retaining fluids and appear heavier.

The best way to measure success is having a body composition analysis done. A popular way is by *bioelectrical impedance*, where a slight electrical impulse is sent through your body to measure the amount of fluid versus fat that's in your body. (Unless you have a pacemaker, bioelectrical impedance is safe. If you're not sure about using bioelectrical impedance, check with your doctor first.) You can even purchase a scale that can do bioelectrical impedance. Body-fat measurement can also be done by an expert using calipers. Or if you have the opportunity to have hydrostatic weighing, it's considered the gold standard of body composition. It's where you are dunked in a big tub of water, expelling all the air you can out of your lungs.

Using the Weight-Loss Log

To monitor your progress, you'll find a Weight-Loss Log in the Appendix, as well as a Body Measurement Log. The Weight-Loss Log works the same way as *The Daily Connection.* You'll be *drawing the line* down through dots to show your progress on a weekly basis. The Body Measurement Log is self-explanatory.

Remember that joke I asked you about earlier, the one about how do you eat an elephant? One bite at a time. The same holds for losing weight. Whether you have 50 pounds or 100 pounds to lose, best you do it gradually and with visuals that are encouraging. It's why the Weight-Loss Log shows only 50 pounds to lose. If you have more than 50 pounds to lose, celebrate your success on this first 50 and then start another Weight-Loss Log.

As you can see in the following example (Figure 17), Eric wanted to lose 45 pounds. His first step was to draw a horizontal line at the number "45". From there, each week when he weighed himself, he drew down through as many dots equal to the number of pounds he lost. Iin his first couple of weeks, he was losing 4 pounds per week. Then it was 3 pounds per week. As is true with any weight-loss approach, things slow down as the body starts readjusting its metabolism. He found himself losing 2 to 2.5 pounds per week thereafter. Things are going just fine for him. Looking at the progress he's made, I'd say by week 8 or 9 he could stop tracking his weight loss. Of course, if he is inspired by the picture he is creating, he certainly could continue *drawing the line* to the finish line "0". Or, if he decides to stop tracking and finds as he weighs himself each week that he is gaining weight, he could pick up where he left off (as you can see with the second "Start Here" arrow).

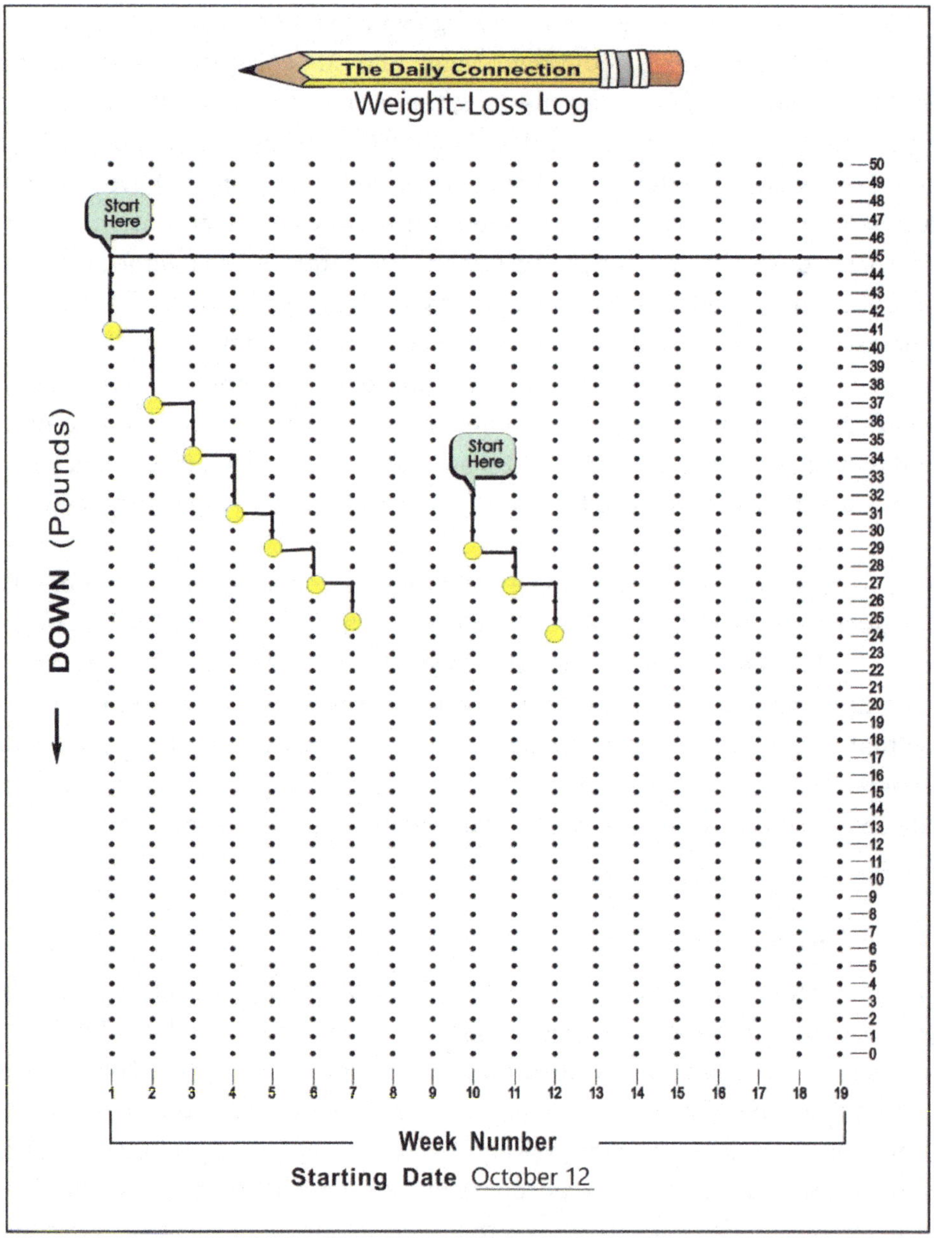

Figure 17

Eric's Weight-Loss Log

Using the Body Measurement Log

As with the Weight-Loss Log, I would suggest you do body measuring once a week. It may come to the point where you needn't do it anymore since your clothes will be telling you what you need to know.

The placement of the tape measure on your body is very important. The "Chest" should be fairly straight-forward, just over the nipples. For the "Waist", place the tape measure right below the rib cage and above the navel. For the "Abdomen", it should be where the stomach protrudes the most. For the "Hips", it should include the largest part of the buttocks. For the "Thighs", it should be where they are the largest.

The log looks like the following:

Date	Chest	Waist	Abdomen	Hips	Thighs

Rewarding Success

Maybe just being successful in accomplishing your goal is enough. Certainly, keeping within the dots on *The Daily Connection* can be rewarding in and of itself. However, there is nothing wrong in physical rewards. I know many people say that when you're trying to lose weight, rewarding yourself with food is wrong. I'm not sure I agree with that. If you've chosen to eliminate some of the higher fat, higher sugar, higher calorie foods to be true to your purpose, then why not celebrate with those foods? One meal does NOT break a good habit you've created. Remember that *Drawing the Line* is really about improving lifestyle habits, not just changing your eating habits.

Now, if you want to avoid using food as a reward, then there's always splurging on a new outfit or two. Heck, you may have to just because your old clothes are too large now. Maybe a spa day would be a nice thing to do for yourself. Or treat yourself with a new something you've been wanting to get but felt a bit guilty for spending the money. Now is as good a time as ever (as long as you don't go bankrupt doing it 😊).

Appendix — WORKSHEETS

The Daily Connection

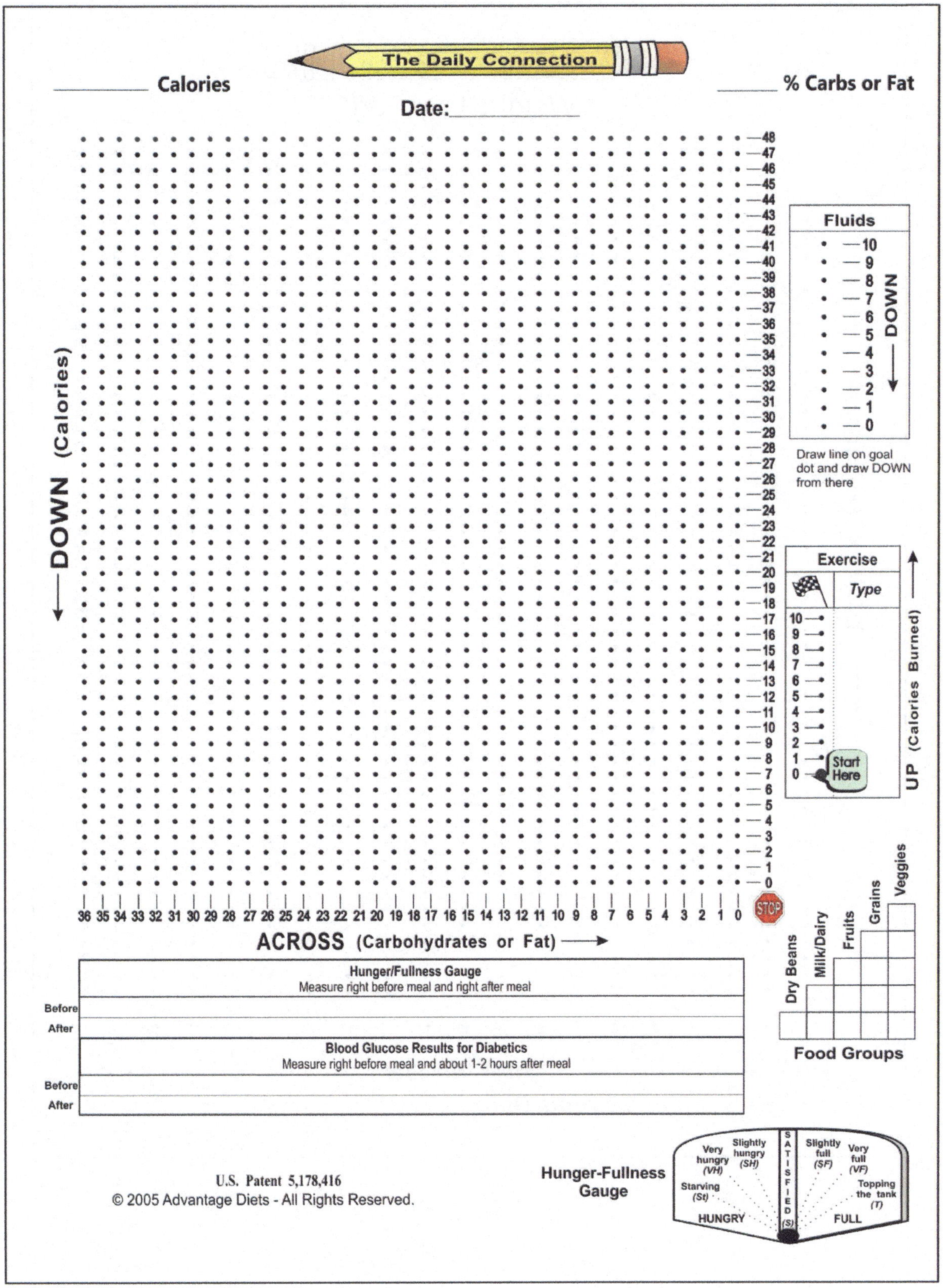

Weight-Loss Log

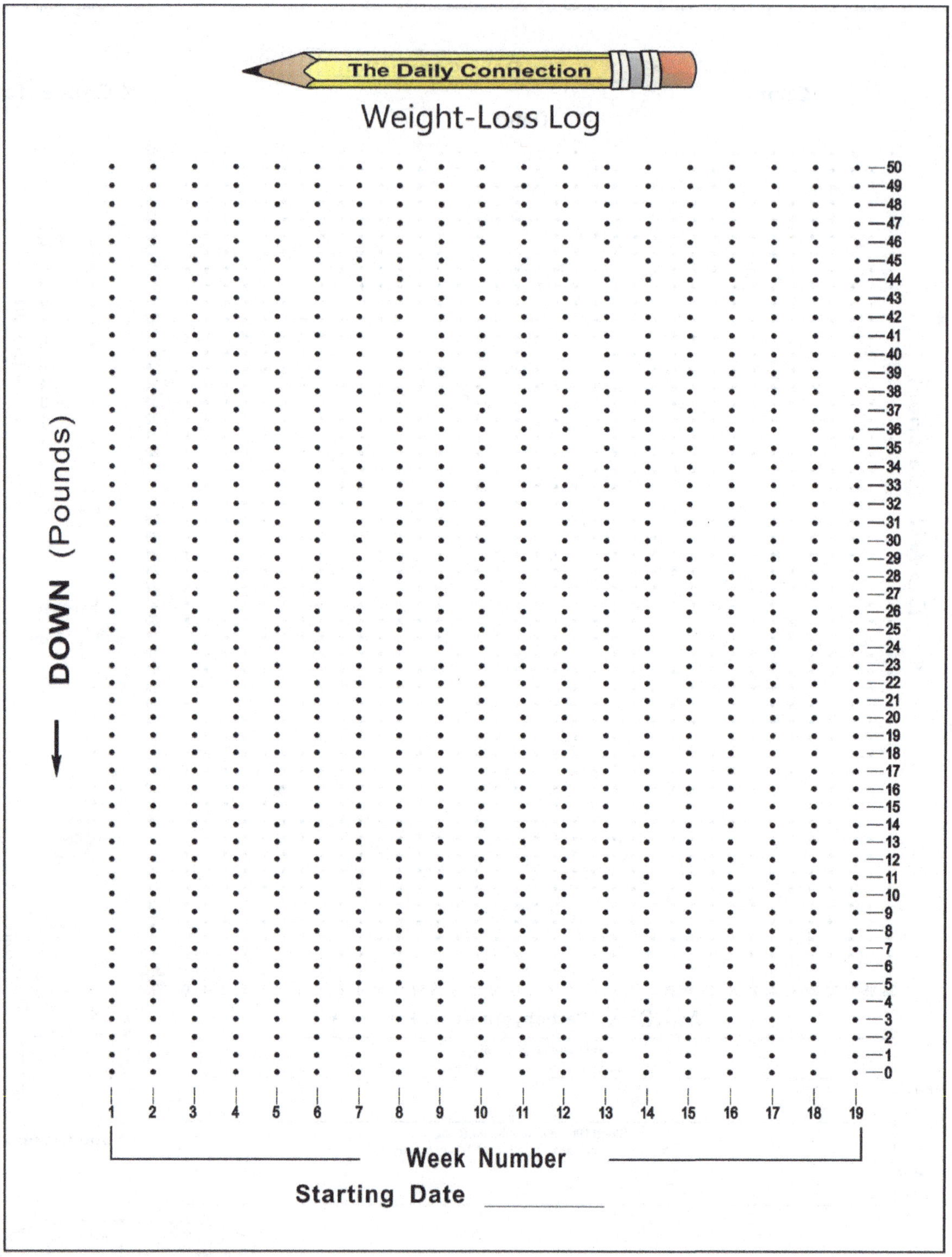

Body Measurement Log

Date	Chest	Waist	Abdomen	Hips	Thighs

Appendix — FOOD LISTS

As discussed earlier in the book, there are four different lists of foods. All the lists contain the same foods. They're just sorted differently as follows:

- The first list is an "Alphabetical" list. You'd use this one when you know what food you want to eat. (Starts on page 59.)
- The second list is of the same foods, except that they are sorted according to the "Least to Most Calories" within each food category and sub-category. This list is handy when you're worried you may go over your calorie allowance for the day. (Starts on page 77.)
- The next list is the "Least to Most Carbohydrates" within each food category and sub-category. Someone counting carbs may find this sorting works well with maintaining a fairly equal distribution of carbohydrates throughout the day. (Starts on page 95.)
- The last list is the "Least to Most Fat" within each food category and sub-category. As the McDonald's example in the book showed (Figure 5), when you've overdone your fat intake for the day and have little to spare for dinner, you can find something that should work with this sorting. (Starts on page 111.)

Even though there are many foods in these lists, still rely on food labels when the information is available to you. It will be the most accurate for that specific food. Consult the Conversion Table on page 14 that shows how to use the numbers you find on the Nutrition Facts Label.

FOOD INDEX	
Category	**Sub-Category**
BEEF	
BEVERAGES	
BREADS	
CAKES	
CANDY	
CEREALS	
CHEESE	
COBBLERS & CRISPS	
COFFEE CAKES, MUFFINS, QUICK BREADS, PANCAKES, & WAFFLES	
CONDIMENTS & SAUCES	
COOKIES	
CRACKERS	
CRUSTS	
CUSTARD & PUDDINGS	
DAIRY	Creamers Milk Sour Cream Yogurt

FOOD INDEX	
Category	**Sub-Category**
EGGS & EGG DISHES	
FAST FOOD	Breakfasts French Fries Salads Sandwiches & Entrees Shakes
FATS	
FISH AND SHELLFISH	Fin Fish Seafood
FRANKS, SAUSAGES, JERKY AND LUNCHEON MEATS	Franks & Sausages Jerky Luncheon Meat
FROZEN DESSERTS	
FRUIT SPREADS & SWEET TOPPINGS	
FRUITS	Canned Dried Fresh
GRAINS	Grains Grain Dishes
LAMB	
MAIN DISHES	Beef Chicken Chinese Italian Japanese Mexican Other Pizza Seafood
NUTS & SEEDS	Nuts Nut butters Seeds (dry roasted)
PIES	
PORK	

FOOD INDEX	
Category	**Sub-Category**
POULTRY	Chicken Turkey Game
SALADS	
SANDWICHES	
SNACKS	
SOUPS	
SWEETENERS	
VEGETABLES — NON-STARCHY	Non-starchy Non-starchy vegetable dishes
VEGETABLES — STARCHY	Beans Corn Green peas Other Potatoes

Food List: Alphabetical

ALPHABETICAL Food	Amt	Calories DOWN	Carbs ACROSS	Fat ACROSS
BEEF (cooked without fat)				
Bottom Round	3 oz	4	0	3
Eye of Round	3 oz	3	0	2
Flank Steak	3 oz	4	0	4
Ground Beef, extra lean	3 oz	3	0	5
Ground Beef, lean	3 oz	5	0	6
Ground Beef, regular	3 oz	5	0	7
Porterhouse	3 oz	5	0	7
Rib Eye	3 oz	5	0	7
Ribs	3 oz	6	0	8
Round	3 oz	4	0	3
Round Tip	3 oz	4	0	3
Short Ribs	3 oz	5	0	7
T-Bone	3 oz	5	0	6
Tenderloin	3 oz	5	0	6
Top Loin	3 oz	4	0	5
Top Round	3 oz	4	0	3
Top Sirloin	3 oz	4	0	4
Veal (ground)	3 oz	3	0	2
Veal Loin	3 oz	4	0	4
Veal Shoulder, Arm	3 oz	3	0	3
BEVERAGES				
ALCOHOL				
Beer	12 fl oz	3	2	0
Distilled spirits (gin, rum, vodka, whiskey, Scotch)	1 fl oz	1	0	0
Liqueurs	1 fl oz	2	2	0
Port	4 fl oz	3	1	0
Red or white wine	4 fl oz	2	0	0
Sherry, Dry	4 fl oz	3	1	0
ESPRESSO (Get Nutrition Facts at coffee shop and convert to dots)				
Tall Latte w/ Nonfat Milk	12 fl oz	2	2	0
Tall Latte w/ Whole Milk	12 fl oz	4	2	4
Tall Mocha w/ Whole Milk	12 fl oz	4	3	3
JUICE and NECTARS				
Apple	8 fl oz	2	3	0
Apricot	8 fl oz	3	4	0
Carrot	8 fl oz	2	3	0
Cranberry Cocktail	8 fl oz	3	4	0
Fruit Punch Drink	8 fl oz	2	4	0
Grape	8 fl oz	3	4	0
Grapefruit	8 fl oz	2	3	0
Lemonade	8 fl oz	2	3	0
Orange	8 fl oz	2	3	0
Papaya	8 fl oz	3	4	0

ALPHABETICAL Food	Amt	Calories DOWN	Carbs ACROSS	Fat ACROSS
BEVERAGES (cont.)				
JUICE and NECTARS (cont.)				
Peach	8 fl oz	3	4	0
Pear	8 fl oz	3	5	0
Prune	8 fl oz	4	5	0
Tomato	8 fl oz	1	1	0
OTHER				
Cocoa	8 fl oz	3	3	0
Eggnog	8 fl oz	7	4	7
Hot Cider	8 fl oz	2	3	0
Milkshake, Vanilla	8 fl oz	5	5	3
Soda	8 fl oz	2	3	0
BREADS				
BAGELS				
All flavors (small)	1	4	5	0
Whole wheat; whole grain (small)	1	4	4	0
BISCUITS, ROLLS, ETC.				
Baking Powder, Buttermilk	1	3	3	3
Bun — Hot dog or Hamburger	1	3	4	0
Corn Pone, Baked	1	3	3	1
Cornbread (2½" square)	1 pc	3	3	1
Crumpet	1	2	2	0
English muffin	1	3	4	0
Roll — Egg dinner	1	2	2	1
Roll — Hawaiian Sweet Bread	1	2	2	1
Roll — Plain (small)	1	2	2	0
Scone	1	3	2	2
OTHER				
Bread sticks (4" x ½")	4	2	2	0
Pita (6" across)	1	3	4	0
Seasoned Croutons, Ready to Eat	¼ cup	1	1	1
Taco Shells	2	2	2	2
Tortilla, corn (6" across)	1	2	2	0
Tortilla, flour (6" across)	1	2	2	0
SLICED BREAD				
Cinnamon, potato, rye, sourdough, white	1 slice	2	2	0
Whole-wheat, whole grain	1 slice	2	1	0
CAKES				
Angel Food Cake (1/12 of cake)	1 slice	3	4	0
Brownie (2" square)	1 pc	3	3	3
Brownie with Chocolate Icing (2" square)	1 pc	4	4	4
Cake with frosting (2½" square)	1 pc	5	4	4
Cake without frosting (2½" square)	1 pc	4	4	2
Carrot Cake (3" square)	1 pc	5	4	5
Cheesecake (1/12 of cake)	1 slice	4	4	10

ALPHABETICAL Food	Amt	Calories DOWN	Carbs ACROSS	Fat ACROSS
CAKES (cont.)				
Cupcake with frosting (small)	1	5	4	4
Doughnut with Creme Filling	1	6	3	6
Doughnut with Jelly Filling	1	6	4	6
Doughnut, Glazed	1	5	3	5
Doughnut, Plain Old Fashioned	1	4	3	5
Fruit Fritter	1	4	3	3
Fruitcake (1" slice)	1 pc	3	3	2
Pineapple Upside Down Cake (2" square)	1 pc	5	4	4
Pound Cake (1½" slice)	1 pc	6	5	5
CANDY				
Almond Paste	2 tbsp	3	2	3
Chocolate Bar with Almonds	1.55 oz	5	5	13
Chocolate Chip Granola Bar	1	4	3	2
Chocolate Fudge	1 oz	3	3	1
Fruit Leather Bar or Roll	1	2	2	0
Hard Candy	2	1	1	0
Jelly Beans	15	3	5	0
Marshmallows	4	2	3	0
Milk Chocolate Bar	3¼ oz	9	6	9
Peanut Brittle	1½ oz	4	4	1
Semi Sweet or Milk Choc Chips	1 oz	3	2	3
CEREALS				
Cereals, cooked	½ cup	2	2	0
Cereals, sweetened, ready-to-eat	½ cup	2	2	0
Cereals, unsweetened, ready-to-eat	¾ cup	2	2	0
Corn Grits, cooked	½ cup	1	2	0
Granola	¼ cup	3	1	3
Granola, low-fat	¼ cup	2	2	1
Puffed Cereal	1½ cups	2	2	0
CHEESE				
American Cheese, Processed	1 oz	2	0	3
Blue Cheese	1 oz	2	0	3
Brie Cheese	1 oz	2	0	3
Cheddar Cheese	1 oz	2	0	4
Cottage Cheese, Low Fat 1%	½ cup	2	0	0
Cottage Cheese, Low Fat 2%	½ cup	2	0	1
Cream Cheese	2 tbsp	2	0	4
Cream Cheese, Fat Free	2 tbsp	1	0	0
Cream Cheese, Light	1 oz	1	0	3
Feta Cheese	1 oz	1	0	2
Gouda Cheese	1 oz	2	0	3
Gruyere Cheese	1 oz	2	0	3
Monterey Jack Cheese	1 oz	2	0	3
Mozzarella Cheese, Part Skim Milk, Low Moisture	1 oz	2	0	2

ALPHABETICAL Food	Amt	Calories DOWN	Carbs ACROSS	Fat ACROSS
CHEESE (cont.)				
Parmesan or Romano Cheese, Grated	2 tbsp	1	0	1
Provolone Cheese	1 oz	2	0	3
Ricotta Cheese, Part Skim Milk	¼ cup	2	0	2
Swiss Cheese	1 oz	2	0	3
COBBLERS & CRISPS				
Fruit Crisp	½ cup	5	6	3
Fruit Cobbler	1 serv	4	5	2
COFFEE CAKES, MUFFINS, QUICK BREADS, PANCAKES, & WAFFLES				
Cinnamon Bun, frosted	1	4	4	3
Coffeecake — cheese, fruit, cinnamon (2½" slice)	1 pc	4	4	3
Danish Pastry, plain	1	4	3	5
French Toast, baked	2 slices	7	5	4
Muffin, cake (small)	1	3	3	2
Pancakes, plain	3	5	4	4
Quick Breads (banana, zucchini, nuts; 1½" slice)	1 pc	3	2	3
Toaster Pastry, fruit	1	4	4	2
Waffle, plain (frozen)	2	4	4	2
CONDIMENTS & SAUCES				
Barbecue Sauce	2 tbsp	1	1	0
Catsup or Ketchup	2 tbsp	1	1	0
Chutney	1 tbsp	1	1	0
Cocktail Sauce	¼ cup	1	2	0
Guacamole	2 tbsp	1	0	2
Hot Dog Pickle Relish	2 tbsp	1	1	0
Mayonnaise	1 tbsp	2	0	3
Mayonnaise, Low calorie	1 tbsp	1	0	1
Mustard	1 tbsp	0	0	0
Olives - large	8 items	1	0	1
Plum Sauce	1 tbsp	1	1	0
Tartar Sauce	2 tbsp	2	0	1
COOKIES				
Animal Crackers	12	3	3	2
Butter cookie	6	3	2	2
Chocolate Chip (1½" across)	1	3	2	3
Chocolate or Vanilla Wafer	5	3	3	2
Fig Bar	2	2	3	1
Fortune cookie	4	2	3	0
Gingersnaps	2	1	1	1
Oatmeal cookie	1	4	3	3
Puffed Rice Cereal and Marshmallow (2" square)	1	2	3	1
Shortbread cookie	4	3	2	3
Sugar cookie (2" across)	2	3	2	2
Vanilla or Chocolate Sandwich with Creme Filling	3	3	2	2

ALPHABETICAL Food	Amt	Calories DOWN	Carbs ACROSS	Fat ACROSS
CRACKERS				
Cheese Cracker Sandwich with Peanut Butter	4	3	2	3
Cheese Crackers	30	3	2	3
Graham Crackers (2½" sq)	4	2	3	1
Matzo Crackers	1	2	3	0
Melba Toast	3	1	1	0
Oyster crackers	20	1	1	1
Rye Crispbread Crackers	1	1	1	0
Saltine Crackers	5	1	1	1
Whole Wheat Crackers	7	2	2	2
CRUSTS				
Graham Cracker Pie Crust	1/8 pie	3	2	3
Pie Crust, Baked	1/8 pie	2	1	3
Pizza Crust	1/8 pie	3	3	1
Vanilla Wafer Pie Crust	1/8 pie	2	1	3
CUSTARD & PUDDINGS				
Gelatin, regular	½ cup	2	2	0
Egg Custard (made with 2% milk)	½ cup	3	3	1
Pudding, regular (made with 2% milk)	½ cup	3	3	1
Pudding, sugar-free (made with 2% milk)	½ cup	2	1	1
Reduced Calorie Gelatin Mix with Aspartame	½ cup	1	1	0
Rice Pudding	½ cup	4	3	2
DAIRY				
CREAM				
Creamer, Non-Dairy, liquid	2 tbsp	1	0	1
Creamer, Non-Dairy, Lite, liquid	2 tbsp	0	0	0
Half and Half	2 tbsp	1	0	1
Heavy, Whipped	2 tbsp	1	0	2
Substitute, Powder	1 tsp	0	0	0
Whipping, Heavy, Liquid	2 tbsp	2	0	4
Whipping, Light, Liquid	2 tbsp	2	0	4
MILK				
1% Low-fat	1 cup	2	1	1
2% Reduced Fat	1 cup	2	1	2
3.3% Whole	1 cup	3	1	3
Nonfat, skim	1 cup	2	1	0
Condensed, sweetened	2 tbsp	2	2	1
Evaporated, whole	2 tbsp	1	0	1
Soy	1 cup	2	1	2

ALPHABETICAL Food	Amt	Calories DOWN	Carbs ACROSS	Fat ACROSS
DAIRY (cont.)				
SOUR CREAM				
Fat Free	2 tbsp	0	1	0
Reduced Fat	2 tbsp	1	0	1
Regular	2 tbsp	1	0	2
YOGURT				
Fruit, Non-Fat, Sweetened with Low Calorie Sweetener	1 cup	2	2	0
Fruit, Low Fat	1 cup	5	6	1
Plain, Non-Fat	1 cup	3	2	0
Plain, Whole Milk	1 cup	3	1	3
EGGS AND EGG DISHES				
Cheese Omelet	1	3	0	4
Egg Omelet	1	2	0	3
Egg Substitute, Liquid	¼ cup	1	0	1
Egg White, Raw	1	0	0	0
Egg Yolk, Raw	3	4	0	6
Egg, Raw	1	1	0	2
Eggs Benedict	1	6	2	7
Scrambled Eggs	¼ cup	2	0	3
Western Omelet with Ham, Onions and Peppers	1	2	0	3
FAST-FOOD				
BREAKFASTS				
Bacon, Egg & Cheese Biscuit	1	9	4	9
Sausage Biscuit with Egg	1	10	4	12
FRENCH FRIES				
Small French Fries	1 order	5	4	4
Medium French Fries	1 order	7	6	6
Large French Fries	1 order	10	8	10
SALADS				
Caesar Salad (without chicken)	1 order	2	1	2
Caesar Salad with Crispy Chicken	1 order	6	3	5
Caesar Salad with Grilled Chicken	1 order	4	1	2
SANDWICHES AND ENTREES				
Cheeseburger	1	6	4	5
Crispy Chicken Pieces	1	10	6	9
Double Cheeseburger	1	9	4	9
Fish Filets	1	8	5	7
Hamburger	1	5	4	3

ALPHABETICAL Food	Amt	Calories DOWN	Carbs ACROSS	Fat ACROSS
FAST-FOOD (cont.)				
SHAKES				
Shake (small)	12 fl oz	9	9	4
Shake (medium)	16 fl oz	12	12	5
Shake (large)	21 fl oz	15	16	7
FATS				
Avocado	½ cup	2	1	4
Butter	1 tbsp	2	0	5
Butter, whipped	1 tbsp	2	0	4
Chicken Fat	1 tbsp	2	0	5
Lard	1 tbsp	2	0	5
Margarine	1 tbsp	2	0	4
Oil: almond. canola, coconut, corn, hazelnut, olive, peanut, safflower, sesame, soybean, sunflower, walnut	1 tbsp	2	0	5
Salad Dressing: Italian	2 tbsp	2	0	3
Salad Dressing: Thousand Island	2 tbsp	2	1	4
Shortening	1 tbsp	2	0	5
FISN AND SHELLFISH (Unless noted, cooked without added fat)				
FIN FISH				
Butterfish	3 oz	3	0	3
Catfish	3 oz	3	0	3
Cod	3 oz	2	0	0
Eel	3 oz	4	0	5
Freshwater Bass	3 oz	2	0	2
Gefilte Fish, Sweet Recipe	3 oz	1	1	1
Halibut	3 oz	2	0	1
Lingcod	3 oz	2	0	0
Mahi Mahi, Dolphinfish or Dorado	3 oz	2	0	0
Monkfish	3 oz	2	0	1
Pollock	3 oz	2	0	0
Pompano	3 oz	4	0	4
Rainbow Trout, Farmed	3 oz	3	0	2
Salmon	3 oz	4	0	4
Surimi	3 oz	2	1	0
Swordfish	2 oz	3	0	2
Tuna, Canned in Water, Drained	2 oz	1	0	0
Whitefish	3 oz	3	0	2
Yellowfin Tuna	3 oz	2	0	0
Swordfish	2 oz	3	0	2
Tuna, Canned in Water, Drained	2 oz	1	0	0
Whitefish	3 oz	3	0	2
Yellowfin Tuna	3 oz	2	0	0

ALPHABETICAL Food	Amt	Calories DOWN	Carbs ACROSS	Fat ACROSS
FISN AND SHELLFISH (cont.)				
SEAFOOD				
Alaska King Crab	3 oz	2	0	1
Blue Mussel	3 oz	3	0	1
Clams	3 oz	3	0	1
Crayfish	3 oz	1	0	0
Dungeness Crab	3 oz	2	0	0
Eastern Oyster	3 oz	1	0	1
Northern Lobster	3 oz	2	0	0
Oysters	3 oz	2	0	2
Scallops	3 oz	2	0	1
Shrimp	3 oz	2	0	0
FRANKS, SAUSAGES, JERKY AND LUNCHEON MEATS				
FRANKS AND SAUSAGES				
Beef and Pork Chorizo	2 oz	5	0	8
Beef and Pork Frankfurter	2 oz	4	0	6
Beef and Pork Knockwurst	2 oz	3	0	6
Beef and Pork Pepperoni	2 oz	6	0	10
Frankfurter, Beef	2 oz	3	0	5
Frankfurter, Chicken	2 oz	2	0	3
Frankfurter, Turkey	2 oz	2	0	3
Pork Bratwurst	2 oz	3	0	6
Pork Sausage Link	2 oz	4	0	7
JERKY				
Beef Jerky	1 oz	2	0	3
Pork Jerky	1 oz	2	0	2
LUNCHEON MEAT				
Bologna, beef	2 oz	4	0	6
Bologna, turkey	1 oz	2	0	3
Corned beef	2 oz	1	0	1
Ham	2 oz	2	0	2
Ham, turkey	2 oz	1	0	1
Pastrami, turkey	2 oz	2	0	1
Prosciutto Ham	2 oz	2	0	2
Roast beef	2 oz	1	0	0
Salami, beef	2 oz	3	0	4
Salami, turkey	2 oz	2	0	3
Turkey breast	1 oz	1	0	0
FROZEN DESSERTS				
Choc Covered Ice Cream Bar	1	3	2	5
Frozen Yogurt, fruit varieties	½ cup	3	3	2
Frozen Yogurt, Vanilla (soft)	½ cup	2	2	2
Ice Cream Sandwich	1	3	3	2
Ice cream, light	½ cup	2	2	1

ALPHABETICAL Food	Amt	Calories DOWN	Carbs ACROSS	Fat ACROSS
FROZEN DESSERTS (cont.)				
Ice cream, regular	½ cup	3	2	3
Ice cream, rich (high fat)	½ cup	6	4	7
Popsicle	1	1	1	0
Sherbet, all flavors	½ cup	3	3	1
FRUIT SPREADS & SWEET TOPPINGS				
Apple Butter	1 tbsp	2	3	0
Chocolate syrup	1 tbsp	1	2	0
Cranberry sauce, jellied	1 tbsp	1	2	0
Honey	1 tbsp	2	2	0
Jam, Jelly or Preserves	1 tbsp	1	2	0
Syrup, light	2 tbsp	2	1	0
Syrup, regular	1 tbsp	2	2	0
FRUITS				
CANNED				
Applesauce, unsweetened	½ cup	1	2	0
Apricots	½ cup	1	2	0
Cherries	½ cup	1	2	0
Fruit cocktail	½ cup	1	2	0
Mandarin Oranges, drained	¾ cup	1	2	0
Peaches	½ cup	1	2	0
Pears	½ cup	1	2	0
Pineapple	½ cup	1	2	0
Plums	½ cup	1	2	0
DRIED				
Apples	4 rings	1	2	0
Apricots	8 halves	1	2	0
Banana Chips	¼ cup	1	2	8
Coconut, sweetened	¼ cup	1	2	8
Dates	3	1	2	0
Figs	2	2	2	0
Prunes	3	1	2	0
Raisins	2 tbsp	1	2	0
FRESH				
Apple, small	1	1	2	0
Apricots	4	1	2	0
Banana, medium	1	2	3	0
Berries (blackberries, blueberries)	¾ cup	1	2	0
Cantaloupe, cubed	1 cup	1	2	0
Cherries	12	1	2	0
Figs, medium	2	1	2	0
Grapefruit	½	1	2	0
Grapes	17	1	2	0
Honeydew, cubed	1 cup	1	2	0
Mango	½	1	2	0
Nectarine, small	1	1	2	0

ALPHABETICAL Food	Amt	Calories DOWN	Carbs ACROSS	Fat ACROSS
FRUITS (cont.)				
FRESH (cont.)				
Orange, small	1	1	2	0
Peaches, medium	1	1	2	0
Pears, small	1	1	2	0
Pineapple	¾ cup	1	2	0
Plums, small	2	1	2	0
Raspberries	1 cup	1	2	0
Strawberries	1¼ cup	1	2	0
Watermelon, cubed	1¼ cup	1	2	0
GRAINS (cooked unless otherwise stated)				
Asian noodles	½ cup	2	2	0
Buckwheat	½ cup	2	2	0
Bulgur	½ cup	2	2	0
Cornmeal (dry)	¼ cup	3	4	1
Couscous	½ cup	2	2	0
Flour (dry)	¼ cup	3	4	0
Grits	½ cup	2	3	0
Millet	½ cup	3	3	0
Pasta - macaroni, spaghetti, linguini, fettuccine, penne, etc.	½ cup	2	2	0
Pearled Barley	½ cup	2	3	0
Potato Gnocchi	½ cup	3	2	3
Ramen Noodles	½ cup	2	2	2
Rice- brown or white	½ cup	3	3	0
GRAIN DISHES				
Rice Pilaf	½ cup	3	3	1
Spanish Rice	½ cup	2	3	1
LAMB (cooked without added fat unless noted)				
Ground	3 oz	5	0	7
Leg	3 oz	5	0	7
Loin	3 oz	5	0	6
Shoulder	3 oz	5	0	6
MAIN DISHES				
BEEF				
Chili Con Carne with Beans	1 cup	6	3	5
Corned Beef Hash	1 cup	8	3	10
Meat Loaf	3 oz	4	1	4
Pot Pie	1 cup	11	5	13
Salisbury Steak	3 oz	4	1	5
Stew with Potatoes, Carrots, Peas and Gravy	1 cup	3	2	1
Stroganoff with Noodles	1 cup	8	4	8
Swedish Meatballs	1 cup	9	4	9
Beef with Noodles in Tomato Sauce	1 cup	6	3	3

ALPHABETICAL Food	Amt	Calories DOWN	Carbs ACROSS	Fat ACROSS
MAIN DISHES (cont.)				
CHICKEN				
Chicken a la King	¾ cup	4	1	2
Fricassee	1 cup	6	1	7
Fried Steak	3 oz	5	1	7
Pot Pie	1 cup	11	5	12
With Barbecue Sauce	5 cups	5	1	5
With Dumplings	1 cup	7	3	7
With Noodles	1 cup	5	3	2
CHINESE				
Beef or Pork Egg Roll	2	5	2	5
Cashew Chicken	1 cup	6	2	7
Chicken and Vegetable Combo	1 cup	6	1	7
Chicken Chow Mein	1 cup	5	1	5
Chop Suey with Beef and Pork	1 cup	6	2	7
Dim Sum with Pork	5	5	2	5
Fried Rice with Meat or Poultry	1 cup	7	5	5
General Tso Chicken	1 cup	6	2	7
Kung Pao Chicken	1 cup	4	1	4
Moo Goo Gai Pan	1 cup	5	1	7
Pork Egg Foo Yung	1	2	0	3
Stir Fried Pork and Vegetables	1 cup	7	0	4
Sweet and Sour Pork	1 cup	5	3	3
ITALIAN				
Chicken or Turkey Cacciatore	5 oz	5	1	6
Chicken or Turkey Tetrazzini	1 cup	7	3	8
Lasagna with Ground Beef	1 cup	6	3	6
Macaroni and Cheese	2/3 cup	7	3	8
Spaghetti and Meat Balls with Tomato Sauce	1 cup	7	5	5
Veal Parmigiana	3 oz	4	1	5
JAPANESE				
Chicken Teriyaki	1 cup	7	2	3
Sushi with Vegetables and Fish	6 pc	4	5	0
MEXICAN				
Bean and Cheese Burrito	1	2	3	2
Bean Burrito	1	7	3	6
Bean Taco or Tostada with Cheese, Lettuce, Tomato, Salsa	2	7	5	6
Beef and Cheese Quesadilla	1	4	2	4
Beef Burrito	1	7	3	8
Beef Taco or Tostada with Cheese, Lettuce, Tomato and Salsa	2	7	3	7
Cheese Enchilada	1	6	3	7
Cheese Quesadilla	1	4	2	4
Chicken Fajita	1	4	1	1

ALPHABETICAL Food	Amt	Calories DOWN	Carbs ACROSS	Fat ACROSS
MAIN DISHES (cont.)				
MEXICAN (cont.)				
Chicken Taco	1	3	2	7
Nachos with Beans and Cheese	1 cup	5	2	5
Pork Tamales	1	4	1	5
Refried Bean and Cheese Burrito, 6-inch Tortilla	1	7	4	6
OTHER				
Cheese Blintzes	2	5	3	5
Cheese Knish	2	8	4	9
Corndog	1	9	7	7
Lamb Stew	1 cup	5	2	2
Pierogi with Potato and Cheese	3	4	4	2
PIZZA				
Cheese	1 slice	6	4	6
Cheese, thick crust	1 slice	8	7	6
Hawaiian	1 slice	7	4	6
Pepperoni	1 slice	7	5	5
SEAFOOD				
Baked Salmon with Cucumber Dill Sauce	1 serv	5	1	3
Bouillabaisse	1 cup	5	1	3
Crab Cakes	1	2	0	2
Fish Fillet, Batter Coated or Breaded, Fried	3 oz	4	2	4
Fish Fillets, baked	3 oz	2	0	0
Japanese Fish Cake Tempura	3 oz	3	1	2
Oysters Rockefeller	1 cup	6	3	7
Paella (Paella a la Marinera)	1 cup	7	3	4
Shrimp, Breaded, Fried	3 oz	4	1	4
Tuna Noodle Casserole with Peas and Mushrooms	1 cup	7	4	5
NUTS AND SEEDS				
NUTS (DRY ROASTED)				
Macadamia nuts	¼ cup	5	1	10
Nuts: almonds, cashews, hazelnuts, peanuts, pistachios	¼ cup	4	1	7
Pecans	¼ cup	4	0	8
Walnuts	¼ cup	4	0	8
NUT BUTTERS				
Almond, Cashew, Peanut Butter, Sesame	2 tbsp	4	1	7
Tahini Butter	2 tbsp	4	1	6
SEEDS (DRY ROASTED)				
Flax Seed	3 tbsp	4	1	5
Sesame Seeds	2 tsp	1	0	1
Sunflower Seed Kernels	¼ cup	4	1	6

ALPHABETICAL Food	**Amt**	**Calories DOWN**	**Carbs ACROSS**	**Fat ACROSS**
PIES				
Custard	1/8 pie	5	4	5
Fruit, 2 crusts	1/8 pie	6	5	5
Lemon Meringue	1/8 pie	7	6	6
Pecan	1/8 pie	9	8	8
Pumpkin	1/8 pie	5	4	4
PORK (cooked without added fat unless noted)				
Bacon	2 slices	2	0	3
Bacon, Canadian style	2 oz	2	0	2
Boston Butt	3 oz	5	0	6
Chop, fried	3 oz	5	1	5
Chop, Center Loin	3 oz	3	0	3
Chop, Top Loin	3 oz	5	0	6
Cured Ham	3 oz	3	0	3
Cutlet	3 oz	5	0	6
Ground	3 oz	6	0	9
Picnic	3 oz	5	0	6
Sausage	3 oz	6	0	9
Shoulder	3 oz	5	0	6
Spareribs	3 oz	6	0	9
Tenderloin	3 oz	3	0	3
POULTRY (Chicken and Turkey) AND GAME (cooked without added fat unless noted)				
CHICKEN				
Breast with skin	3 oz	3	0	3
Breast, Fried	3 oz	4	0	3
Breast, skinless	3 oz	3	0	1
Leg with skin	3 oz	4	0	4
Leg, Fried	3 oz	4	0	5
Leg, skinless	3 oz	3	0	3
Thigh with skin	3 oz	5	0	5
Thigh, Fried	3 oz	4	0	5
Thigh, skinless	3 oz	4	0	4
Wing, Fried	3 oz	5	0	7
Wing	3 oz	5	0	6
TURKEY				
Breast with skin	3 oz	3	0	2
Dark Meat with skin	3 oz	4	0	4
Ground Turkey	3 oz	4	0	4
Leg with skin	3 oz	4	0	3
Light Meat with skin	3 oz	3	0	3
Light Meat, skinless	3 oz	3	0	1

ALPHABETICAL Food	Amt	Calories DOWN	Carbs ACROSS	Fat ACROSS
POULTRY (Chicken and Turkey) AND GAME (cont.)				
GAME				
Cornish Game Hen with skin	3 oz	5	0	6
Deer or Venison Chops	3 oz	4	0	3
Duck with skin	3 oz	6	0	9
Goose with skin	3 oz	5	0	7
Rabbit	3 oz	3	0	3
SALADS				
Caesar Salad with Dressing	1 cup	3	1	5
Carrot Raisin Salad	½ cup	4	2	6
Chef Salad with Turkey, Ham and Cheese	¾ cup	3	0	3
Cobb Salad with Dressing	1 cup	4	1	6
Coleslaw	¾ cup	1	1	1
Macaroni Salad	½ cup	4	2	4
Potato Salad	½ cup	4	2	5
Tabouli, Tabbouleh or Tabouli	1 cup	4	2	6
SANDWICHES				
Bacon and Egg Croissant	1	8	4	10
Bacon, Lettuce and Tomato with Mayonnaise	1	7	4	7
Bologna with Margarine	1	5	3	5
Breaded Chicken Fillet with Lettuce, Tomato and Mayonnaise	1	8	4	10
Broiled Chicken Fillet on Whole Wheat Roll with Lettuce, Tomato and Mayonnaise	1	7	4	3
Cheeseburger, 1/4 lb. with Mayonnaise and Tomatoes	1	11	5	13
Chicken Salad Spread	1	7	3	6
Chili Hot Dog with Bun	1	7	3	8
Corned Beef	1	5	3	4
Egg Salad	1	6	3	5
Grilled Cheese	1	6	3	6
Ham and Cheese	1	7	4	6
Hot Dog on Bun	1	5	2	6
Meatball and Spaghetti Sauce Submarine on Roll	1	9	4	8
Pastrami	1	7	3	7
Peanut Butter and Jelly	1	7	5	6
Roast Beef Submarine with Mayonnaise and Vegetables	1	8	5	5
Tuna Salad	1	8	3	9
Turkey Submarine with Cheese, Lettuce, Tomato and Mayonnaise – 6"	1	5	5	3

ALPHABETICAL Food	Amt	Calories DOWN	Carbs ACROSS	Fat ACROSS
SNACKS				
Bagel Chips	½ cup	2	3	1
Corn Chips	1 oz	3	2	4
Popcorn, Air Popped	3 ¾ cup	2	3	0
Popcorn, Caramel	1 cup	3	3	2
Popcorn, Popped in Oil	3 cups	3	2	4
Potato Chips, baked	1 oz	2	3	1
Potato Chips, light	1 oz	3	2	2
Pretzel Sticks, Thin	10	2	2	0
Pretzel, Soft	1	4	5	1
Pretzel, Whole Wheat	1 oz	2	3	0
Rice cakes	2	1	2	0
Taro Chips	1 oz	3	2	3
Tortilla Chips	1 oz	3	2	3
Tortilla Chips, baked	1 oz	1	3	0
Tortilla Chips, light	1 oz	3	2	2
Trail Mix	¼ cup	3	2	4
SOUPS				
Beef or Chicken Noodle	1 cup	2	1	1
Bird's Nest with Chicken, Ham, Noodles	1 cup	2	1	1
Black Bean	1 cup	2	2	1
Chicken Broth	1 cup	1	0	1
Chunky Bean with Ham	1 cup	5	2	3
Chunky Chicken Noodle	1 cup	4	2	2
Chunky Minestrone	1 cup	3	2	1
Chunky Potato Ham Chowder	1 cup	4	2	5
Cream of Asparagus (made with Milk)	1 cup	3	2	3
Cream of Mushroom (made with milk)	1 cup	4	2	5
Cream of Potato (made with milk)	1 cup	3	2	2
Green Pea Soup (made with milk)	1 cup	5	4	3
Lentil and Ham	1 cup	3	2	1
Manhattan Clam Chowder	1 cup	3	2	1
Onion Soup	1 cup	1	1	1
Oyster Stew (made with milk)	1 cup	3	1	3
Ramen Noodle	1 cup	3	2	3
Split Pea with Ham	1 cup	4	3	2
Tomato (made with milk)	1 cup	3	3	2
Vegetable Beef	1 cup	2	1	1

ALPHABETICAL Food	Amt	Calories DOWN	Carbs ACROSS	Fat ACROSS
SWEETENERS				
Honey	1 tbsp	1	2	0
Molasses	1 tbsp	1	2	0
Powdered Sugar	3 tbsp	1	1	0
White Granulated Sugar	3 tbsp	1	1	0
VEGETABLES – Non-Starchy				
Generally, ½ cup cooked or 1 cup raw equals one serving. If DOWN is "0" and you eat two servings, count DOWN as 1 Dot				
Artichoke Hearts, cooked	½ cup	1	1	0
Asparagus, cooked	½ cup	0	0	0
Beans: Yellow, Green, String or Wax, cooked	2/3 cup	1	1	0
Beets, sliced, Canned	½ cup	1	1	0
Bell or Sweet Pepper, cooked	½ cup	0	0	0
Broccoli Spears, cooked	½ cup	1	1	0
Brussels Sprouts, cooked	½ cup	1	1	0
Cabbage (cooked): Green, Napa, Red, Savoy	½ cup	0	0	0
Carrots, cooked	2/3 cup	1	1	0
Cauliflower, cooked	½ cup	0	0	0
Celery Stalk	2	0	0	0
Cucumber, sliced	¾ cup	0	0	0
Eggplant, cooked	1 cup	1	1	0
Greens (cooked): Beet, Collards, Kale, Mustard, Spinach, Swiss Chard	½ cup	0	0	0
Leeks, cooked	¾ cup	0	1	0
Mushrooms, cooked	½ cup	0	0	0
Onions, Chopped	¾ cup	0	1	0
Salad Greens: Butterhead, Boston, Bibb, Endive, Escarole, Iceberg, Spinach	1½ cups	0	0	0
Snow or Sugar Peas, cooked	½ cup	1	1	0
Tomato	1	1	1	0
Tomato Puree, Canned	¼ cup	1	1	0
Watercress	1 cup	0	0	0
Zucchini Summer Squash, cooked	½ cup	0	0	0
VEGETABLE DISHES				
Onion Rings, Breaded and Pan Fried	11	6	4	8
Vegetable Tempura	12 pc	3	2	5

ALPHABETICAL Food	Amt	Calories DOWN	Carbs ACROSS	Fat ACROSS
VEGETABLES —Starchy				
BEANS				
Baked Beans	½ cup	4	3	1
Blackeye, garbanzo, kidney, lentils, lima, navy, pinto, Split pea	½ cup	2	1	0
Refried	½ cup	2	2	1
Soybeans, boiled	½ cup	3	0	3
CORN				
White Hominy	½ cup	1	1	0
White, Yellow, or Creamed	½ cup	2	3	0
GREEN PEAS				
Green Peas	½ cup	1	1	0
Green Peas and Carrots	½ cup	1	1	0
OTHER				
Hummus	½ cup	4	2	4
Jerusalem Artichoke	½ cup	1	2	0
Parsnips	½ cup	1	2	0
Pumpkin Pie Mix, Canned	½ cup	3	4	0
Tofu	½ cup	2	0	2
Winter Squash, All Varieties, Baked, Mashed	2/3 cup	1	1	0
POTATOES				
Au Gratin	½ cup	3	2	3
Baked	1	5	5	7
French Fried, Hashed Brown	½ cup	3	2	4
Mashed	2/3 cup	3	3	2
Orange Glazed Yams	¼ cup	3	3	1
Scalloped	½ cup	2	2	1
Sweet or Yam	¾ cup	2	3	0

Food List: Least to Most Calories

LEAST TO MOST CALORIES Food	Amt	Calories DOWN	Carbs ACROSS	Fat ACROSS
BEEF (cooked without fat)				
Eye of Round	3 oz	3	0	2
Ground Beef, extra lean	3 oz	3	0	5
Veal (ground)	3 oz	3	0	2
Veal Shoulder, Arm	3 oz	3	0	3
Bottom Round	3 oz	4	0	3
Flank Steak	3 oz	4	0	4
Round	3 oz	4	0	3
Round Tip	3 oz	4	0	3
Top Loin	3 oz	4	0	5
Top Round	3 oz	4	0	3
Top Sirloin	3 oz	4	0	4
Veal Loin	3 oz	4	0	4
Ground Beef, lean	3 oz	5	0	6
Ground Beef, regular	3 oz	5	0	7
Porterhouse	3 oz	5	0	7
Rib Eye	3 oz	5	0	7
Short Ribs	3 oz	5	0	7
T-Bone	3 oz	5	0	6
Tenderloin	3 oz	5	0	6
Ribs	3 oz	6	0	8
BEVERAGES				
ALCOHOL				
Distilled spirits (gin, rum, vodka, whiskey, Scotch)	1 fl oz	1	0	0
Liqueurs	1 fl oz	2	2	0
Red or white wine	4 fl oz	2	0	0
Beer	12 fl oz	3	2	0
Port	4 fl oz	3	1	0
Sherry, Dry	4 fl oz	3	1	0
ESPRESSO (Get Nutrition Facts at coffee shop and convert to dots)				
Tall Latte w/ Nonfat Milk	12 fl oz	2	2	0
Tall Latte w/ Whole Milk	12 fl oz	4	2	4
Tall Mocha w/ Whole Milk	12 fl oz	4	3	3
JUICE and NECTARS				
Tomato	8 fl oz	1	1	0
Apple	8 fl oz	2	3	0
Carrot	8 fl oz	2	3	0
Fruit Punch Drink	8 fl oz	2	4	0
Grapefruit	8 fl oz	2	3	0
Lemonade	8 fl oz	2	3	0
Orange	8 fl oz	2	3	0
Apricot	8 fl oz	3	4	0
Cranberry Cocktail	8 fl oz	3	4	0
Grape	8 fl oz	3	4	0

LEAST TO MOST CALORIES Food	Amt	Calories DOWN	Carbs ACROSS	Fat ACROSS
BEVERAGES (cont.)				
JUICE and NECTARS (cont.)				
Papaya	8 fl oz	3	4	0
Peach	8 fl oz	3	4	0
Pear	8 fl oz	3	5	0
Prune	8 fl oz	4	5	0
OTHER				
Hot Cider	8 fl oz	2	3	0
Soda	8 fl oz	2	3	0
Cocoa	8 fl oz	3	3	0
Milkshake, Vanilla	8 fl oz	5	5	3
Eggnog	8 fl oz	7	4	7
BREADS				
BAGELS				
All flavors (small)	1	4	5	0
Whole wheat; whole grain (small)	1	4	4	0
BISCUITS, ROLLS, ETC.				
Crumpet	1	2	2	0
Roll — Egg dinner	1	2	2	1
Roll — Hawaiian Sweet Bread	1	2	2	1
Roll — Plain (small)	1	2	2	0
Baking Powder, Buttermilk	1	3	3	3
Bun — Hot dog or Hamburger	1	3	4	0
Corn Pone, Baked	1	3	3	1
Cornbread (2½" square)	1 pc	3	3	1
English muffin	1	3	4	0
Scone	1	3	2	2
OTHER				
Seasoned Croutons, Ready to Eat	¼ cup	1	1	1
Bread sticks (4" x ½")	4	2	2	0
Taco Shells	2	2	2	2
Tortilla, corn (6" across)	1	2	2	0
Tortilla, flour (6" across)	1	2	2	0
Pita (6" across)	1	3	4	0
SLICED BREAD				
Cinnamon, potato, rye, sourdough, white	1 slice	2	2	0
Whole-wheat, whole grain	1 slice	2	1	0
CAKES				
Angel Food Cake (1/12 of cake)	1 slice	3	4	0
Fruitcake (1" slice)	1 pc	3	3	2
Brownie (2" square)	1 pc	3	3	3
Brownie with Chocolate Icing (2" square)	1 pc	4	4	4
Cake without frosting (2½" square)	1 pc	4	4	2
Cheesecake (1/12 of cake)	1 slice	4	4	10
Doughnut, Plain Old Fashioned	1	4	3	5

LEAST TO MOST CALORIES Food	Amt	Calories DOWN	Carbs ACROSS	Fat ACROSS
CAKES (cont.)				
Fruit Fritter	1	4	3	3
Cake with frosting (2½" square)	1 pc	5	4	4
Carrot Cake (3" square)	1 pc	5	4	5
Cupcake with frosting (small)	1	5	4	4
Doughnut, Glazed	1	5	3	5
Pineapple Upside Down Cake (2" square)	1 pc	5	4	4
Doughnut with Creme Filling	1	6	3	6
Doughnut with Jelly Filling	1	6	4	6
Pound Cake (1½" slice)	1 pc	6	5	5
CANDY				
Hard Candy	2	1	1	0
Fruit Leather Bar or Roll	1	2	2	0
Marshmallows	4	2	3	0
Almond Paste	2 tbsp	3	2	3
Chocolate Fudge	1 oz	3	3	1
Jelly Beans	15	3	5	0
Semi Sweet or Milk Choc Chips	1 oz	3	2	3
Chocolate Chip Granola Bar	1	4	3	2
Peanut Brittle	1½ oz	4	4	1
Milk Chocolate Bar	1.55 oz	5	3	5
Chocolate Bar with Almonds	1.55 oz	5	3	5
CEREALS				
Corn Grits, cooked	½ cup	1	2	0
Cereals, cooked	½ cup	2	2	0
Cereals, sweetened, ready-to-eat	½ cup	2	2	0
Cereals, unsweetened, ready-to-eat	¾ cup	2	2	0
Granola, low-fat	¼ cup	2	2	1
Puffed Cereal	1½ cups	2	2	0
Granola	¼ cup	3	1	3
CHEESE				
Cream Cheese, Fat Free	2 tbsp	1	0	0
Cream Cheese, Light	1 oz	1	0	3
Feta Cheese	1 oz	1	0	2
Parmesan or Romano Cheese, Grated	2 tbsp	1	0	1
American Cheese, Processed	1 oz	2	0	3
Blue Cheese	1 oz	2	0	3
Brie Cheese	1 oz	2	0	3
Cheddar Cheese	1 oz	2	0	4
Cottage Cheese, Low Fat 1%	½ cup	2	0	0
Cottage Cheese, Low Fat 2%	½ cup	2	0	1
Cream Cheese	2 tbsp	2	0	4
Gouda Cheese	1 oz	2	0	3
Gruyere Cheese	1 oz	2	0	3
Monterey Jack Cheese	1 oz	2	0	3
Mozzarella Cheese, Part Skim Milk, Low moisture	1 oz	2	0	2

LEAST TO MOST CALORIES Food	Amt	Calories DOWN	Carbs ACROSS	Fat ACROSS
CHEESE (cont.)				
Provolone Cheese	1 oz	2	0	3
Ricotta Cheese, Part Skim Milk	¼ cup	2	0	2
Swiss Cheese	1 oz	2	0	3
COBBLERS & CRISPS				
Fruit Cobbler	1 serv	4	5	2
Fruit Crisp	½ cup	5	6	3
COFFEE CAKES, MUFFINS, QUICK BREADS, PANCAKES, & WAFFLES				
Muffin, cake (small)	1	3	3	2
Quick Breads (banana, zucchini, nuts; 1½" slice)	1 pc	3	2	3
Cinnamon Bun, frosted	1	4	4	3
Coffeecake — cheese, fruit, cinnamon (2½" slice)	1 pc	4	4	3
Danish Pastry, plain	1	4	3	5
Toaster Pastry, fruit	1	4	4	2
Waffle, plain (frozen)	2	4	4	2
Pancakes, plain	3	5	4	4
French Toast, baked	2 slices	7	5	4
CONDIMENTS & SAUCES				
Mustard	1 tbsp	0	0	0
Barbecue Sauce	2 tbsp	1	1	0
Catsup or Ketchup	2 tbsp	1	1	0
Chutney	1 tbsp	1	1	0
Cocktail Sauce	¼ cup	1	2	0
Guacamole	2 tbsp	1	0	2
Hot Dog Pickle Relish	2 tbsp	1	1	0
Mayonnaise, Low calorie	1 tbsp	1	0	1
Olives - large	8 items	1	0	1
Plum Sauce	1 tbsp	1	1	0
Mayonnaise	1 tbsp	2	0	3
Tartar Sauce	2 tbsp	2	0	1
COOKIES				
Gingersnaps	2	1	1	1
Fig Bar	2	2	3	1
Fortune cookie	4	2	3	0
Puffed Rice Cereal and Marshmallow (2" square)	1	2	3	1
Animal Crackers	12	3	3	2
Butter cookie	6	3	2	2
Chocolate Chip (1½" across)	1	3	2	3
Chocolate or Vanilla Wafer	5	3	3	2
Shortbread cookie	4	3	2	3
Sugar cookie (2" across)	2	3	2	2
Vanilla or Chocolate Sandwich with Creme Filling	3	3	2	2
Oatmeal cookie	1	4	3	3

LEAST TO MOST CALORIES Food	Amt	Calories DOWN	Carbs ACROSS	Fat ACROSS
CRACKERS				
Melba Toast	3	1	1	0
Oyster crackers	20	1	1	1
Rye Crispbread Crackers	1	1	1	0
Saltine Crackers	5	1	1	1
Graham Crackers (2½" sq)	4	2	3	1
Matzo Crackers	1	2	3	0
Whole Wheat Crackers	7	2	2	2
Cheese Cracker Sandwich with Peanut Butter	4	3	2	3
Cheese Crackers	30	3	2	3
CRUSTS				
Pie Crust, Baked	1/8 pie	2	1	3
Vanilla Wafer Pie Crust	1/8 pie	2	1	3
Graham Cracker Pie Crust	1/8 pie	3	2	3
Pizza Crust	1/8 pie	3	3	1
CUSTARD & PUDDINGS				
Reduced Calorie Gelatin Mix with Aspartame	½ cup	1	1	0
Gelatin, regular	½ cup	2	2	0
Pudding, sugar-free (made with 2% milk)	½ cup	2	1	1
Egg Custard (made with 2% milk)	½ cup	3	3	1
Pudding, regular (made with 2% milk)	½ cup	3	3	1
Rice Pudding	½ cup	4	3	2
DAIRY				
CREAM				
Creamer, Non-Dairy, Lite, liquid	2 tbsp	0	0	0
Substitute, Powder	1 tsp	0	0	0
Creamer, Non-Dairy, liquid	2 tbsp	1	0	1
Half and Half	2 tbsp	1	0	1
Heavy, Whipped	2 tbsp	1	0	2
Whipping, Heavy, Liquid	2 tbsp	2	0	4
Whipping, Light, Liquid	2 tbsp	2	0	4
MILK				
Evaporated, whole	2 tbsp	1	0	1
1% Low-fat	1 cup	2	1	1
2% Reduced Fat	1 cup	2	1	2
Nonfat, skim	1 cup	2	1	0
Condensed, sweetened	2 tbsp	2	2	1
Soy	1 cup	2	1	2
3.3% Whole	1 cup	3	1	3

LEAST TO MOST CALORIES Food	Amt	Calories DOWN	Carbs ACROSS	Fat ACROSS
DAIRY (cont.)				
SOUR CREAM				
Fat Free	2 tbsp	0	1	0
Reduced Fat	2 tbsp	1	0	1
Regular	2 tbsp	1	0	2
YOGURT				
Fruit, Non-Fat, Sweetened with Low Calorie Sweetener	1 cup	2	2	0
Plain, Non-Fat	1 cup	3	2	0
Plain, Whole Milk	1 cup	3	1	3
Fruit, Low Fat	1 cup	5	6	1
EGGS AND EGG DISHES				
Egg White, Raw	1	0	0	0
Egg Substitute, Liquid	¼ cup	1	0	1
Egg, Raw	1	1	0	2
Egg Omelet	1	2	0	3
Scrambled Eggs	¼ cup	2	0	3
Western Omelet with Ham, Onions and Peppers	1	2	0	3
Cheese Omelet	1	3	0	4
Egg Yolk, Raw	3	4	0	6
Eggs Benedict	1	6	2	7
FAST-FOOD				
BREAKFASTS				
Bacon, Egg & Cheese Biscuit	1	9	4	9
Sausage Biscuit with Egg	1	10	4	12
FRENCH FRIES				
Small French Fries	1 order	5	4	4
Medium French Fries	1 order	7	6	6
Large French Fries	1 order	10	8	10
SALADS				
Caesar Salad (without chicken)	1 order	2	1	2
Caesar Salad with Grilled Chicken	1 order	4	1	2
Caesar Salad with Crispy Chicken	1 order	6	3	5
SANDWICHES AND ENTREES				
Hamburger	1	5	4	3
Cheeseburger	1	6	4	5
Fish Filets	1	8	5	7
Double Cheeseburger	1	9	4	9
Crispy Chicken Pieces	1	10	6	9

LEAST TO MOST CALORIES Food	Amt	Calories DOWN	Carbs ACROSS	Fat ACROSS
FAST-FOOD (cont.)				
SHAKES				
Shake (small)	12 fl oz	9	9	4
Shake (medium)	16 fl oz	12	12	5
Shake (large)	21 fl oz	15	16	7
FATS				
Avocado	½ cup	2	1	4
Butter	1 tbsp	2	0	5
Butter, whipped	1 tbsp	2	0	4
Chicken Fat	1 tbsp	2	0	5
Lard	1 tbsp	2	0	5
Margarine	1 tbsp	2	0	4
Oil: almond. canola, coconut, corn, hazelnut, olive, peanut, safflower, sesame, soybean, sunflower, walnut	1 tbsp	2	0	5
Salad Dressing: Italian	2 tbsp	2	0	3
Salad Dressing: Thousand Island	2 tbsp	2	1	4
Shortening	1 tbsp	2	0	5
FISN AND SHELLFISH (Unless noted, cooked without added fat)				
FIN FISH				
Gefilte Fish, Sweet Recipe	3 oz	1	1	1
Tuna, Canned in Water, Drained	2 oz	1	0	0
Tuna, Canned in Water, Drained	2 oz	1	0	0
Cod	3 oz	2	0	0
Freshwater Bass	3 oz	2	0	2
Halibut	3 oz	2	0	1
Lingcod	3 oz	2	0	0
Mahi Mahi, Dolphinfish or Dorado	3 oz	2	0	0
Monkfish	3 oz	2	0	1
Pollock	3 oz	2	0	0
Surimi	3 oz	2	1	0
Yellowfin Tuna	3 oz	2	0	0
Yellowfin Tuna	3 oz	2	0	0
Butterfish	3 oz	3	0	3
Catfish	3 oz	3	0	3
Rainbow Trout, Farmed	3 oz	3	0	2
Swordfish	2 oz	3	0	2
Whitefish	3 oz	3	0	2
Swordfish	2 oz	3	0	2
Whitefish	3 oz	3	0	2
Eel	3 oz	4	0	5
Pompano	3 oz	4	0	4
Salmon	3 oz	4	0	4

LEAST TO MOST CALORIES Food	Amt	Calories DOWN	Carbs ACROSS	Fat ACROSS
FISN AND SHELLFISH (cont.)				
SEAFOOD				
Crayfish	3 oz	1	0	0
Eastern Oyster	3 oz	1	0	1
Alaska King Crab	3 oz	2	0	1
Dungeness Crab	3 oz	2	0	0
Northern Lobster	3 oz	2	0	0
Oysters	3 oz	2	0	2
Scallops	3 oz	2	0	1
Shrimp	3 oz	2	0	0
Blue Mussel	3 oz	3	0	1
Clams	3 oz	3	0	1
FRANKS, SAUSAGES, JERKY AND LUNCHEON MEATS				
FRANKS AND SAUSAGES				
Frankfurter, Chicken	2 oz	2	0	3
Frankfurter, Turkey	2 oz	2	0	3
Beef and Pork Knockwurst	2 oz	3	0	6
Frankfurter, Beef	2 oz	3	0	5
Pork Bratwurst	2 oz	3	0	6
Beef and Pork Frankfurter	2 oz	4	0	6
Pork Sausage Link	2 oz	4	0	7
Beef and Pork Chorizo	2 oz	5	0	8
Beef and Pork Pepperoni	2 oz	6	0	10
JERKY				
Beef Jerky	1 oz	2	0	3
Pork Jerky	1 oz	2	0	2
LUNCHEON MEAT				
Corned beef	2 oz	1	0	1
Ham, turkey	2 oz	1	0	1
Roast beef	2 oz	1	0	0
Turkey breast	1 oz	1	0	0
Bologna, turkey	1 oz	2	0	3
Ham	2 oz	2	0	2
Pastrami, turkey	2 oz	2	0	1
Prosciutto Ham	2 oz	2	0	2
Salami, turkey	2 oz	2	0	3
Salami, beef	2 oz	3	0	4
Bologna, beef	2 oz	4	0	6
FROZEN DESSERTS				
Popsicle	1	1	1	0
Frozen Yogurt, Vanilla (soft)	½ cup	2	2	2
Ice cream, light	½ cup	2	2	1
Choc Covered Ice Cream Bar	1	3	2	5
Frozen Yogurt, fruit varieties	½ cup	3	3	2

LEAST TO MOST CALORIES Food	Amt	Calories DOWN	Carbs ACROSS	Fat ACROSS
FROZEN DESSERTS (cont.)				
Ice Cream Sandwich	1	3	3	2
Ice cream, regular	½ cup	3	2	3
Sherbet, all flavors	½ cup	3	3	1
Ice cream, rich (high fat)	½ cup	6	4	7
FRUIT SPREADS & SWEET TOPPINGS				
Chocolate syrup	1 tbsp	1	2	0
Cranberry sauce, jellied	1 tbsp	1	2	0
Jam, Jelly or Preserves	1 tbsp	1	2	0
Apple Butter	1 tbsp	2	3	0
Honey	1 tbsp	2	2	0
Syrup, light	2 tbsp	2	1	0
Syrup, regular	1 tbsp	2	2	0
FRUITS				
CANNED				
Applesauce, unsweetened	½ cup	1	2	0
Apricots	½ cup	1	2	0
Cherries	½ cup	1	2	0
Fruit cocktail	½ cup	1	2	0
Mandarin Oranges, drained	¾ cup	1	2	0
Peaches	½ cup	1	2	0
Pears	½ cup	1	2	0
Pineapple	½ cup	1	2	0
Plums	½ cup	1	2	0
DRIED				
Apples	4 rings	1	2	0
Apricots	8 halves	1	2	0
Banana Chips	¼ cup	1	2	8
Coconut, sweetened	¼ cup	1	2	8
Dates	3	1	2	0
Prunes	3	1	2	0
Raisins	2 tbsp	1	2	0
Figs	2	2	2	0
FRESH				
Apple, small	1	1	2	0
Apricots	4	1	2	0
Berries (blackberries, blueberries)	¾ cup	1	2	0
Cantaloupe, cubed	1 cup	1	2	0
Cherries	12	1	2	0
Figs, medium	2	1	2	0
Grapefruit	½	1	2	0
Grapes	17	1	2	0
Honeydew, cubed	1 cup	1	2	0
Mango	½	1	2	0
Nectarine, small	1	1	2	0

LEAST TO MOST CALORIES Food	Amt	Calories DOWN	Carbs ACROSS	Fat ACROSS
FRUITS (cont.)				
FRESH (cont.)				
Orange, small	1	1	2	0
Peaches, medium	1	1	2	0
Pears, small	1	1	2	0
Pineapple	¾ cup	1	2	0
Plums, small	2	1	2	0
Raspberries	1 cup	1	2	0
Strawberries	1¼ cup	1	2	0
Watermelon, cubed	1¼ cup	1	2	0
Banana, medium	1	2	3	0
GRAINS (cooked unless otherwise stated)				
Asian noodles	½ cup	2	2	0
Buckwheat	½ cup	2	2	0
Bulgur	½ cup	2	2	0
Couscous	½ cup	2	2	0
Grits	½ cup	2	3	0
Pasta - macaroni, spaghetti, linguini, fettuccine, penne, etc.	½ cup	2	2	0
Pearled Barley	½ cup	2	3	0
Ramen Noodles	½ cup	2	2	2
Cornmeal (dry)	¼ cup	3	4	1
Flour (dry)	¼ cup	3	4	0
Millet	½ cup	3	3	0
Potato Gnocchi	½ cup	3	2	3
Rice- brown or white	½ cup	3	3	0
GRAIN DISHES				
Spanish Rice	½ cup	2	3	1
Rice Pilaf	½ cup	3	3	1
LAMB (cooked without added fat unless noted)				
Ground	3 oz	5	0	7
Leg	3 oz	5	0	7
Loin	3 oz	5	0	6
Shoulder	3 oz	5	0	6
MAIN DISHES				
BEEF				
Stew with Potatoes, Carrots, Peas and Gravy	1 cup	3	2	1
Meat Loaf	3 oz	4	1	4
Salisbury Steak	3 oz	4	1	5
Chili Con Carne with Beans	1 cup	6	3	5
Beef with Noodles in Tomato Sauce	1 cup	6	3	3
Corned Beef Hash	1 cup	8	3	10
Stroganoff with Noodles	1 cup	8	4	8
Swedish Meatballs	1 cup	9	4	9
Pot Pie	1 cup	11	5	13

LEAST TO MOST CALORIES Food	Amt	Calories DOWN	Carbs ACROSS	Fat ACROSS
MAIN DISHES (cont.)				
CHICKEN				
Chicken a la King	¾ cup	4	1	2
Fried Steak	3 oz	5	1	7
With Barbecue Sauce	5 cups	5	1	5
With Noodles	1 cup	5	3	2
Fricassee	1 cup	6	1	7
With Dumplings	1 cup	7	3	7
Pot Pie	1 cup	11	5	12
CHINESE				
Pork Egg Foo Yung	1	2	0	3
Kung Pao Chicken	1 cup	4	1	4
Beef or Pork Egg Roll	2	5	2	5
Chicken Chow Mein	1 cup	5	1	5
Dim Sum with Pork	5	5	2	5
Moo Goo Gai Pan	1 cup	5	1	7
Sweet and Sour Pork	1 cup	5	3	3
Chicken and Vegetable Combo	1 cup	6	1	7
Chop Suey with Beef and Pork	1 cup	6	2	7
General Tso Chicken	1 cup	6	2	7
Cashew Chicken	1 cup	6	2	7
Fried Rice with Meat or Poultry	1 cup	7	5	5
Stir Fried Pork and Vegetables	1 cup	7	0	4
ITALIAN				
Veal Parmigiana	3 oz	4	1	5
Chicken or Turkey Cacciatore	5 oz	5	1	6
Lasagna with Ground Beef	1 cup	6	3	6
Chicken or Turkey Tetrazzini	1 cup	7	3	8
Macaroni and Cheese	2/3 cup	7	3	8
Spaghetti and Meat Balls with Tomato Sauce	1 cup	7	5	5
JAPANESE				
Sushi with Vegetables and Fish	6 pc	4	5	0
Chicken Teriyaki	1 cup	7	2	3
MEXICAN				
Bean and Cheese Burrito	1	2	3	2
Chicken Taco	1	3	2	7
Beef and Cheese Quesadilla	1	4	2	4
Cheese Quesadilla	1	4	2	4
Chicken Fajita	1	4	1	1
Pork Tamales	1	4	1	5
Nachos with Beans and Cheese	1 cup	5	2	5
Cheese Enchilada	1	6	3	7
Bean Burrito	1	7	3	6
Bean Taco or Tostada with Cheese, Lettuce, Tomato, Salsa	2	7	5	6

LEAST TO MOST CALORIES Food	Amt	Calories DOWN	Carbs ACROSS	Fat ACROSS
MAIN DISHES (cont.)				
MEXICAN (cont.)				
Beef Burrito	1	7	3	8
Beef Taco or Tostada with Cheese, Lettuce, Tomato and Salsa	2	7	3	7
Refried Bean and Cheese Burrito, 6-inch Tortilla	1	7	4	6
OTHER				
Pierogi with Potato and Cheese	3	4	4	2
Cheese Blintzes	2	5	3	5
Lamb Stew	1 cup	5	2	2
Cheese Knish	2	8	4	9
Corndog	1	9	7	7
PIZZA				
Cheese	1 slice	6	4	6
Hawaiian	1 slice	7	4	6
Pepperoni	1 slice	7	5	5
Cheese, thick crust	1 slice	8	7	6
SEAFOOD				
Crab Cakes	1	2	0	2
Fish Fillets, baked	3 oz	2	0	0
Japanese Fish Cake Tempura	3 oz	3	1	2
Fish Fillet, Batter Coated or Breaded, Fried	3 oz	4	2	4
Shrimp, Breaded, Fried	3 oz	4	1	4
Baked Salmon with Cucumber Dill Sauce	1 serv	5	1	3
Bouillabaisse	1 cup	5	1	3
Oysters Rockefeller	1 cup	6	3	7
Paella (Paella a la Marinera)	1 cup	7	3	4
Tuna Noodle Casserole with Peas and Mushrooms	1 cup	7	4	5
NUTS AND SEEDS				
NUTS (DRY ROASTED)				
Nuts: almonds, cashews, hazelnuts, peanuts, pistachios	¼ cup	4	1	7
Pecans	¼ cup	4	0	8
Walnuts	¼ cup	4	0	8
Macadamia nuts	¼ cup	5	1	10
NUT BUTTERS				
Almond, Cashew, Peanut Butter, Sesame	2 tbsp	4	1	7
Tahini Butter	2 tbsp	4	1	6
SEEDS (DRY ROASTED)				
Sesame Seeds	2 tsp	1	0	1
Flax Seed	3 tbsp	4	1	5
Sunflower Seed Kernels	¼ cup	4	1	6

LEAST TO MOST CALORIES Food	Amt	Calories DOWN	Carbs ACROSS	Fat ACROSS
PIES				
Custard	1/8 pie	5	4	5
Pumpkin	1/8 pie	5	4	4
Fruit, 2 crusts	1/8 pie	6	5	5
Lemon Meringue	1/8 pie	7	6	6
Pecan	1/8 pie	9	8	8
PORK (cooked without added fat unless noted)				
Bacon	2 slices	2	0	3
Bacon, Canadian style	2 oz	2	0	2
Chop, Center Loin	3 oz	3	0	3
Cured Ham	3 oz	3	0	3
Tenderloin	3 oz	3	0	3
Boston Butt	3 oz	5	0	6
Chop, fried	3 oz	5	1	5
Chop, Top Loin	3 oz	5	0	6
Cutlet	3 oz	5	0	6
Picnic	3 oz	5	0	6
Shoulder	3 oz	5	0	6
Ground	3 oz	6	0	9
Sausage	3 oz	6	0	9
Spareribs	3 oz	6	0	9
POULTRY (Chicken and Turkey) AND GAME (cooked without added fat unless noted)				
CHICKEN				
Breast with skin	3 oz	3	0	3
Breast, skinless	3 oz	3	0	1
Leg, skinless	3 oz	3	0	3
Breast, Fried	3 oz	4	0	3
Leg with skin	3 oz	4	0	4
Leg, Fried	3 oz	4	0	5
Thigh, Fried	3 oz	4	0	5
Thigh, skinless	3 oz	4	0	4
Thigh with skin	3 oz	5	0	5
Wing, Fried	3 oz	5	0	7
Wing	3 oz	5	0	6
TURKEY				
Breast with skin	3 oz	3	0	2
Light Meat with skin	3 oz	3	0	3
Light Meat, skinless	3 oz	3	0	1
Dark Meat with skin	3 oz	4	0	4
Ground Turkey	3 oz	4	0	4
Leg with skin	3 oz	4	0	3

LEAST TO MOST CALORIES Food	Amt	Calories DOWN	Carbs ACROSS	Fat ACROSS
POULTRY (Chicken and Turkey) AND GAME (cont.)				
GAME				
Rabbit	3 oz	3	0	3
Deer or Venison Chops	3 oz	4	0	3
Cornish Game Hen with skin	3 oz	5	0	6
Goose with skin	3 oz	5	0	7
Duck with skin	3 oz	6	0	9
SALADS				
Coleslaw	¾ cup	1	1	1
Caesar Salad with Dressing	1 cup	3	1	5
Chef Salad with Turkey, Ham and Cheese	¾ cup	3	0	3
Carrot Raisin Salad	½ cup	4	2	6
Cobb Salad with Dressing	1 cup	4	1	6
Macaroni Salad	½ cup	4	2	4
Potato Salad	½ cup	4	2	5
Tabouli, Tabbouleh or Tabouli	1 cup	4	2	6
SANDWICHES				
Bologna with Margarine	1	5	3	5
Corned Beef	1	5	3	4
Hot Dog on Bun	1	5	2	6
Turkey Submarine with Cheese, Lettuce, Tomato and Mayonnaise -6"	1	5	5	3
Egg Salad	1	6	3	5
Grilled Cheese	1	6	3	6
Bacon, Lettuce and Tomato with Mayonnaise	1	7	4	7
Broiled Chicken Fillet on Whole Wheat Roll with Lettuce, Tomato and Mayonnaise	1	7	4	3
Chicken Salad Spread	1	7	3	6
Chili Hot Dog with Bun	1	7	3	8
Ham and Cheese	1	7	4	6
Pastrami	1	7	3	7
Peanut Butter and Jelly	1	7	5	6
Bacon and Egg Croissant	1	8	4	10
Roast Beef Submarine with Mayonnaise and Vegetables	1	8	5	5
Tuna Salad	1	8	3	9
Breaded Chicken Fillet with Lettuce, Tomato and Mayonnaise	1	8	4	10
Meatball and Spaghetti Sauce Submarine on Roll	1	9	4	8
Cheeseburger, 1/4 lb. with Mayonnaise and Tomatoes	1	11	5	13

LEAST TO MOST CALORIES Food	Amt	Calories DOWN	Carbs ACROSS	Fat ACROSS
SNACKS				
Rice cakes	2	1	2	0
Tortilla Chips, baked	1 oz	1	3	0
Bagel Chips	½ cup	2	3	1
Popcorn, Air Popped	3 ¾ cup	2	3	0
Potato Chips, baked	1 oz	2	3	1
Pretzel Sticks, Thin	10	2	2	0
Pretzel, Whole Wheat	1 oz	2	3	0
Corn Chips	1 oz	3	2	4
Popcorn, Caramel	1 cup	3	3	2
Popcorn, Popped in Oil	3 cups	3	2	4
Potato Chips, light	1 oz	3	2	2
Taro Chips	1 oz	3	2	3
Tortilla Chips	1 oz	3	2	3
Tortilla Chips, light	1 oz	3	2	2
Trail Mix	¼ cup	3	2	4
Pretzel, Soft	1	4	5	1
SOUPS				
Chicken Broth	1 cup	1	0	1
Onion Soup	1 cup	1	1	1
Beef or Chicken Noodle	1 cup	2	1	1
Bird's Nest with Chicken, Ham, Noodles	1 cup	2	1	1
Black Bean	1 cup	2	2	1
Vegetable Beef	1 cup	2	1	1
Chunky Minestrone	1 cup	3	2	1
Cream of Asparagus (made with Milk)	1 cup	3	2	3
Cream of Potato (made with milk)	1 cup	3	2	2
Lentil and Ham	1 cup	3	2	1
Manhattan Clam Chowder	1 cup	3	2	1
Oyster Stew (made with milk)	1 cup	3	1	3
Ramen Noodle	1 cup	3	2	3
Tomato (made with milk)	1 cup	3	3	2
Chunky Chicken Noodle	1 cup	4	2	2
Chunky Potato Ham Chowder	1 cup	4	2	5
Cream of Mushroom (made with milk)	1 cup	4	2	5
Split Pea with Ham	1 cup	4	3	2
Chunky Bean with Ham	1 cup	5	2	3
Green Pea Soup (made with milk)	1 cup	5	4	3

LEAST TO MOST CALORIES Food	Amt	Calories DOWN	Carbs ACROSS	Fat ACROSS
SWEETENERS				
Honey	1 tbsp	1	2	0
Molasses	1 tbsp	1	2	0
Powdered Sugar	3 tbsp	1	1	0
White Granulated Sugar	3 tbsp	1	1	0
VEGETABLES – Non-Starchy				
Generally, ½ cup cooked or 1 cup raw equals one serving. If DOWN is "0" and you eat two servings, count DOWN as 1 Dot				
Asparagus, cooked	½ cup	0	0	0
Bell or Sweet Pepper, cooked	½ cup	0	0	0
Cabbage (cooked): Green, Napa, Red, Savoy	½ cup	0	0	0
Cauliflower, cooked	½ cup	0	0	0
Celery Stalk	2	0	0	0
Cucumber, sliced	¾ cup	0	0	0
Greens (cooked): Beet, Collards, Kale, Mustard, Spinach, Swiss Chard	½ cup	0	0	0
Leeks, cooked	¾ cup	0	1	0
Mushrooms, cooked	½ cup	0	0	0
Onions, Chopped	¾ cup	0	1	0
Salad Greens: Butterhead, Boston, Bibb, Endive, Escarole, Iceberg, Spinach	1½ cups	0	0	0
Watercress	1 cup	0	0	0
Zucchini Summer Squash, cooked	½ cup	0	0	0
Artichoke Hearts, cooked	½ cup	1	1	0
Beans: Yellow, Green, String or Wax, cooked	2/3 cup	1	1	0
Beets, sliced, Canned	½ cup	1	1	0
Broccoli Spears, cooked	½ cup	1	1	0
Brussels Sprouts, cooked	½ cup	1	1	0
Carrots, cooked	2/3 cup	1	1	0
Eggplant, cooked	1 cup	1	1	0
Snow or Sugar Peas, cooked	½ cup	1	1	0
Tomato	1	1	1	0
Tomato Puree, Canned	¼ cup	1	1	0
VEGETABLE DISHES				
Vegetable Tempura	12 pc	3	2	5
Onion Rings, Breaded and Pan Fried	11	6	4	8

LEAST TO MOST CALORIES Food	Amt	Calories DOWN	Carbs ACROSS	Fat ACROSS
VEGETABLES —Starchy				
BEANS				
Blackeye, garbanzo, kidney, lentils, lima, navy, pinto, Split pea	½ cup	2	1	0
Refried	½ cup	2	2	1
Soybeans, boiled	½ cup	3	0	3
Baked Beans	½ cup	4	3	1
CORN				
White Hominy	½ cup	1	1	0
White, Yellow, or Creamed	½ cup	2	3	0
GREEN PEAS				
Green Peas	½ cup	1	1	0
Green Peas and Carrots	½ cup	1	1	0
OTHER				
Jerusalem Artichoke	½ cup	1	2	0
Parsnips	½ cup	1	2	0
Winter Squash, All Varieties, Baked, Mashed	2/3 cup	1	1	0
Tofu	½ cup	2	0	2
Pumpkin Pie Mix, Canned	½ cup	3	4	0
Hummus	½ cup	4	2	4
POTATOES				
Scalloped	½ cup	2	2	1
Sweet or Yam	¾ cup	2	3	0
Au Gratin	½ cup	3	2	3
French Fried, Hashed Brown	½ cup	3	2	4
Mashed	2/3 cup	3	3	2
Orange Glazed Yams	¼ cup	3	3	1
Baked	1	5	5	7

Food List: Least to Most Carbohydrates

LEAST TO MOST CARBOHYDRATES Food	Amt	Calories DOWN	Carbs ACROSS	Fat ACROSS
BEEF (cooked without fat)				
Bottom Round	3 oz	4	0	3
Eye of Round	3 oz	3	0	2
Flank Steak	3 oz	4	0	4
Ground Beef, extra lean	3 oz	3	0	5
Ground Beef, lean	3 oz	5	0	6
Ground Beef, regular	3 oz	5	0	7
Porterhouse	3 oz	5	0	7
Rib Eye	3 oz	5	0	7
Ribs	3 oz	6	0	8
Round	3 oz	4	0	3
Round Tip	3 oz	4	0	3
Short Ribs	3 oz	5	0	7
T-Bone	3 oz	5	0	6
Tenderloin	3 oz	5	0	6
Top Loin	3 oz	4	0	5
Top Round	3 oz	4	0	3
Top Sirloin	3 oz	4	0	4
Veal (ground)	3 oz	3	0	2
Veal Loin	3 oz	4	0	4
Veal Shoulder, Arm	3 oz	3	0	3
BEVERAGES				
ALCOHOL				
Distilled spirits (gin, rum, vodka, whiskey, Scotch)	1 fl oz	1	0	0
Red or white wine	4 fl oz	2	0	0
Port	4 fl oz	3	1	0
Sherry, Dry	4 fl oz	3	1	0
Beer	12 fl oz	3	2	0
Liqueurs	1 fl oz	2	2	0
ESPRESSO (Get Nutrition Facts at coffee shop and convert to dots)				
Tall Latte w/ Nonfat Milk	12 fl oz	2	2	0
Tall Latte w/ Whole Milk	12 fl oz	4	2	4
Tall Mocha w/ Whole Milk	12 fl oz	4	3	3
JUICE and NECTARS				
Tomato	8 fl oz	1	1	0
Apple	8 fl oz	2	3	0
Carrot	8 fl oz	2	3	0
Grapefruit	8 fl oz	2	3	0
Lemonade	8 fl oz	2	3	0
Orange	8 fl oz	2	3	0
Apricot	8 fl oz	3	4	0
Cranberry Cocktail	8 fl oz	3	4	0
Fruit Punch Drink	8 fl oz	2	4	0
Grape	8 fl oz	3	4	0

LEAST TO MOST CARBOHYDRATES Food	Amt	Calories DOWN	Carbs ACROSS	Fat ACROSS
BEVERAGES (cont.)				
JUICE and NECTARS (cont.)				
Papaya	8 fl oz	3	4	0
Peach	8 fl oz	3	4	0
Pear	8 fl oz	3	5	0
Prune	8 fl oz	4	5	0
OTHER				
Cocoa	8 fl oz	3	3	0
Hot Cider	8 fl oz	2	3	0
Soda	8 fl oz	2	3	0
Eggnog	8 fl oz	7	4	7
Milkshake, Vanilla	8 fl oz	5	5	3
BREADS				
BAGELS				
Whole wheat; whole grain (small)	1	4	4	0
All flavors (small)	1	4	5	0
BISCUITS, ROLLS, ETC.				
Crumpet	1	2	2	0
Roll — Egg dinner	1	2	2	1
Roll — Hawaiian Sweet Bread	1	2	2	1
Roll — Plain (small)	1	2	2	0
Scone	1	3	2	2
Baking Powder, Buttermilk	1	3	3	3
Corn Pone, Baked	1	3	3	1
Cornbread (2½" square)	1 pc	3	3	1
Bun — Hot dog or Hamburger	1	3	4	0
English muffin	1	3	4	0
OTHER				
Seasoned Croutons, Ready to Eat	¼ cup	1	1	1
Bread sticks (4" x ½ ")	4	2	2	0
Taco Shells	2	2	2	2
Tortilla, corn (6" across)	1	2	2	0
Tortilla, flour (6" across)	1	2	2	0
Pita (6" across)	1	3	4	0
SLICED BREAD				
Whole-wheat, whole grain	1 slice	2	1	0
Cinnamon, potato, rye, sourdough, white	1 slice	2	2	0
CAKES				
Brownie (2" square)	1 pc	3	3	3
Angel Food Cake (1/12 of cake)	1 slice	3	4	0
Brownie with Chocolate Icing (2" square)	1 pc	4	4	4
Cake with frosting (2½" square)	1 pc	5	4	4
Cake without frosting (2½" square)	1 pc	4	4	2
Carrot Cake (3" square)	1 pc	5	4	5
Cheesecake (1/12 of cake)	1 slice	4	4	10

LEAST TO MOST CARBOHYDRATES Food	Amt	Calories DOWN	Carbs ACROSS	Fat ACROSS
CAKES (cont.)				
Doughnut with Creme Filling	1	6	3	6
Doughnut, Glazed	1	5	3	5
Doughnut, Plain Old Fashioned	1	4	3	5
Fruit Fritter	1	4	3	3
Fruitcake (1" slice)	1 pc	3	3	2
Cupcake with frosting (small)	1	5	4	4
Doughnut with Jelly Filling	1	6	4	6
Pineapple Upside Down Cake (2" square)	1 pc	5	4	4
Pound Cake (1½" slice)	1 pc	6	5	5
CANDY				
Hard Candy	2	1	1	0
Fruit Leather Bar or Roll	1	2	2	0
Almond Paste	2 tbsp	3	2	3
Semi Sweet or Milk Choc Chips	1 oz	3	2	3
Marshmallows	4	2	3	0
Chocolate Fudge	1 oz	3	3	1
Chocolate Chip Granola Bar	1	4	3	2
Chocolate Bar with Almonds	3 oz	5	3	5
Milk Chocolate Bar	3¼ oz	5	3	5
Peanut Brittle	1½ oz	4	4	1
Jelly Beans	15	3	5	0
CEREALS				
Granola	¼ cup	3	1	3
Cereals, cooked	½ cup	2	2	0
Cereals, sweetened, ready-to-eat	½ cup	2	2	0
Cereals, unsweetened, ready-to-eat	¾ cup	2	2	0
Corn Grits, cooked	½ cup	1	2	0
Granola, low-fat	¼ cup	2	2	1
Puffed Cereal	1½ cups	2	2	0
CHEESE				
American Cheese, Processed	1 oz	2	0	3
Blue Cheese	1 oz	2	0	3
Brie Cheese	1 oz	2	0	3
Cheddar Cheese	1 oz	2	0	4
Cottage Cheese, Low Fat 1%	½ cup	2	0	0
Cottage Cheese, Low Fat 2%	½ cup	2	0	1
Cream Cheese	2 tbsp	2	0	4
Cream Cheese, Fat Free	2 tbsp	1	0	0
Cream Cheese, Light	1 oz	1	0	3
Feta Cheese	1 oz	1	0	2
Gouda Cheese	1 oz	2	0	3
Gruyere Cheese	1 oz	2	0	3
Monterey Jack Cheese	1 oz	2	0	3
Mozzarella Cheese, Part Skim Milk, Low Moisture	1 oz	2	0	2

LEAST TO MOST CARBOHYDRATES Food	Amt	Calories DOWN	Carbs ACROSS	Fat ACROSS
CHEESE (cont.)				
Parmesan or Romano Cheese, Grated	2 tbsp	1	0	1
Provolone Cheese	1 oz	2	0	3
Ricotta Cheese, Part Skim Milk	¼ cup	2	0	2
Swiss Cheese	1 oz	2	0	3
COBBLERS & CRISPS				
Fruit Cobbler	1 serv	4	5	2
Fruit Crisp	½ cup	5	6	3
COFFEE CAKES, MUFFINS, QUICK BREADS, PANCAKES, & WAFFLES				
Quick Breads (banana, zucchini, nuts; 1½" slice)	1 pc	3	2	3
Danish Pastry, plain	1	4	3	5
Muffin, cake (small)	1	3	3	2
Cinnamon Bun, frosted	1	4	4	3
Coffeecake — cheese, fruit, cinnamon (2½" slice)	1 pc	4	4	3
Pancakes, plain	3	5	4	4
Toaster Pastry, fruit	1	4	4	2
Waffle, plain (frozen)	2	4	4	2
French Toast, baked	2 slices	7	5	4
CONDIMENTS & SAUCES				
Guacamole	2 tbsp	1	0	2
Mayonnaise	1 tbsp	2	0	3
Mayonnaise, Low calorie	1 tbsp	1	0	1
Mustard	1 tbsp	0	0	0
Olives - large	8 items	1	0	1
Tartar Sauce	2 tbsp	2	0	1
Barbecue Sauce	2 tbsp	1	1	0
Catsup or Ketchup	2 tbsp	1	1	0
Chutney	1 tbsp	1	1	0
Hot Dog Pickle Relish	2 tbsp	1	1	0
Plum Sauce	1 tbsp	1	1	0
Cocktail Sauce	¼ cup	1	2	0
COOKIES				
Gingersnaps	2	1	1	1
Butter cookie	6	3	2	2
Chocolate Chip (1½" across)	1	3	2	3
Shortbread cookie	4	3	2	3
Sugar cookie (2" across)	2	3	2	2
Vanilla or Chocolate Sandwich with Creme Filling	3	3	2	2
Animal Crackers	12	3	3	2
Chocolate or Vanilla Wafer	5	3	3	2
Fig Bar	2	2	3	1
Fortune cookie	4	2	3	0
Oatmeal cookie	1	4	3	3
Puffed Rice Cereal and Marshmallow (2" square)	1	2	3	1

LEAST TO MOST CARBOHYDRATES Food	Amt	Calories DOWN	Carbs ACROSS	Fat ACROSS
CRACKERS				
Melba Toast	3	1	1	0
Oyster crackers	20	1	1	1
Rye Crispbread Crackers	1	1	1	0
Saltine Crackers	5	1	1	1
Cheese Cracker Sandwich with Peanut Butter	4	3	2	3
Cheese Crackers	30	3	2	3
Whole Wheat Crackers	7	2	2	2
Graham Crackers (2½" sq)	4	2	3	1
Matzo Crackers	1	2	3	0
CRUSTS				
Pie Crust, Baked	1/8 pie	2	1	3
Vanilla Wafer Pie Crust	1/8 pie	2	1	3
Graham Cracker Pie Crust	1/8 pie	3	2	3
Pizza Crust	1/8 pie	3	3	1
CUSTARD & PUDDINGS				
Pudding, sugar-free (made with 2% milk)	½ cup	2	1	1
Reduced Calorie Gelatin Mix with Aspartame	½ cup	1	1	0
Gelatin, regular	½ cup	2	2	0
Egg Custard (made with 2% milk)	½ cup	3	3	1
Pudding, regular (made with 2% milk)	½ cup	3	3	1
Rice Pudding	½ cup	4	3	2
DAIRY				
CREAM				
Creamer, Non-Dairy, liquid	2 tbsp	1	0	1
Creamer, Non-Dairy, Lite, liquid	2 tbsp	0	0	0
Half and Half	2 tbsp	1	0	1
Heavy, Whipped	2 tbsp	1	0	2
Substitute, Powder	1 tsp	0	0	0
Whipping, Heavy, Liquid	2 tbsp	2	0	4
Whipping, Light, Liquid	2 tbsp	2	0	4
MILK				
Evaporated, whole	2 tbsp	1	0	1
1% Low-fat	1 cup	2	1	1
2% Reduced Fat	1 cup	2	1	2
3.3% Whole	1 cup	3	1	3
Nonfat, skim	1 cup	2	1	0
Soy	1 cup	2	1	2
Condensed, sweetened	2 tbsp	2	2	1

LEAST TO MOST CARBOHYDRATES Food	Amt	Calories DOWN	Carbs ACROSS	Fat ACROSS
DAIRY (cont.)				
SOUR CREAM				
Reduced Fat	2 tbsp	1	0	1
Regular	2 tbsp	1	0	2
Fat Free	2 tbsp	0	1	0
YOGURT				
Plain, Whole Milk	1 cup	3	1	3
Fruit, Non-Fat, Sweetened with Low Calorie Sweetener	1 cup	2	2	0
Plain, Non-Fat	1 cup	3	2	0
Fruit, Low Fat	1 cup	5	6	1
EGGS AND EGG DISHES				
Cheese Omelet	1	3	0	4
Egg Omelet	1	2	0	3
Egg Substitute, Liquid	¼ cup	1	0	1
Egg White, Raw	1	0	0	0
Egg Yolk, Raw	3	4	0	6
Egg, Raw	1	1	0	2
Scrambled Eggs	¼ cup	2	0	3
Western Omelet with Ham, Onions and Peppers	1	2	0	3
Eggs Benedict	1	6	2	7
FAST-FOOD				
BREAKFASTS				
Bacon, Egg & Cheese Biscuit	1	9	4	9
Sausage Biscuit with Egg	1	10	4	12
FRENCH FRIES				
Small French Fries	1 order	5	4	4
Medium French Fries	1 order	7	6	6
Large French Fries	1 order	10	8	10
SALADS				
Caesar Salad (without chicken)	1 order	2	1	2
Caesar Salad with Grilled Chicken	1 order	4	1	2
Caesar Salad with Crispy Chicken	1 order	6	3	5
SANDWICHES AND ENTREES				
Cheeseburger	1	6	4	5
Double Cheeseburger	1	9	4	9
Hamburger	1	5	4	3
Fish Filets	1	8	5	7
Crispy Chicken Pieces	1	10	6	9

LEAST TO MOST CARBOHYDRATES Food	Amt	Calories DOWN	Carbs ACROSS	Fat ACROSS
FAST-FOOD (cont.)				
SHAKES				
Shake (small)	12 fl oz	9	9	4
Shake (medium)	16 fl oz	12	12	5
Shake (large)	21 fl oz	15	16	7
FATS				
Butter	1 tbsp	2	0	5
Butter, whipped	1 tbsp	2	0	4
Chicken Fat	1 tbsp	2	0	5
Lard	1 tbsp	2	0	5
Margarine	1 tbsp	2	0	4
Oil: almond. canola, coconut, corn, hazelnut, olive, peanut, safflower, sesame, soybean, sunflower, walnut	1 tbsp	2	0	5
Salad Dressing: Italian	2 tbsp	2	0	3
Shortening	1 tbsp	2	0	5
Avocado	½ cup	2	1	4
Salad Dressing: Thousand Island	2 tbsp	2	1	4
FISN AND SHELLFISH (Unless noted, cooked without added fat)				
FIN FISH				
Butterfish	3 oz	3	0	3
Catfish	3 oz	3	0	3
Cod	3 oz	2	0	0
Eel	3 oz	4	0	5
Freshwater Bass	3 oz	2	0	2
Halibut	3 oz	2	0	1
Lingcod	3 oz	2	0	0
Mahi Mahi, Dolphinfish or Dorado	3 oz	2	0	0
Monkfish	3 oz	2	0	1
Pollock	3 oz	2	0	0
Pompano	3 oz	4	0	4
Rainbow Trout, Farmed	3 oz	3	0	2
Salmon	3 oz	4	0	4
Swordfish	2 oz	3	0	2
Tuna, Canned in Water, Drained	2 oz	1	0	0
Whitefish	3 oz	3	0	2
Yellowfin Tuna	3 oz	2	0	0
Swordfish	2 oz	3	0	2
Tuna, Canned in Water, Drained	2 oz	1	0	0
Whitefish	3 oz	3	0	2
Yellowfin Tuna	3 oz	2	0	0
Gefilte Fish, Sweet Recipe	3 oz	1	1	1
Surimi	3 oz	2	1	0

LEAST TO MOST CARBOHYDRATES Food	Amt	Calories DOWN	Carbs ACROSS	Fat ACROSS
FISN AND SHELLFISH (cont.)				
SEAFOOD				
Alaska King Crab	3 oz	2	0	1
Blue Mussel	3 oz	3	0	1
Clams	3 oz	3	0	1
Crayfish	3 oz	1	0	0
Dungeness Crab	3 oz	2	0	0
Eastern Oyster	3 oz	1	0	1
Northern Lobster	3 oz	2	0	0
Oysters	3 oz	2	0	2
Scallops	3 oz	2	0	1
Shrimp	3 oz	2	0	0
FRANKS, SAUSAGES, JERKY AND LUNCHEON MEATS				
FRANKS AND SAUSAGES				
Beef and Pork Chorizo	2 oz	5	0	8
Beef and Pork Frankfurter	2 oz	4	0	6
Beef and Pork Knockwurst	2 oz	3	0	6
Beef and Pork Pepperoni	2 oz	6	0	10
Frankfurter, Beef	2 oz	3	0	5
Frankfurter, Chicken	2 oz	2	0	3
Frankfurter, Turkey	2 oz	2	0	3
Pork Bratwurst	2 oz	3	0	6
Pork Sausage Link	2 oz	4	0	7
JERKY				
Beef Jerky	1 oz	2	0	3
Pork Jerky	1 oz	2	0	2
LUNCHEON MEAT				
Bologna, beef	2 oz	4	0	6
Bologna, turkey	1 oz	2	0	3
Corned beef	2 oz	1	0	1
Ham	2 oz	2	0	2
Ham, turkey	2 oz	1	0	1
Pastrami, turkey	2 oz	2	0	1
Prosciutto Ham	2 oz	2	0	2
Roast beef	2 oz	1	0	0
Salami, beef	2 oz	3	0	4
Salami, turkey	2 oz	2	0	3
Turkey breast	1 oz	1	0	0
FROZEN DESSERTS				
Popsicle	1	1	1	0
Choc Covered Ice Cream Bar	1	3	2	5
Frozen Yogurt, Vanilla (soft)	½ cup	2	2	2
Ice cream, light	½ cup	2	2	1
Ice cream, regular	½ cup	3	2	3

LEAST TO MOST CARBOHYDRATES Food	Amt	Calories DOWN	Carbs ACROSS	Fat ACROSS
FROZEN DESSERTS (cont.)				
Frozen Yogurt, fruit varieties	½ cup	3	3	2
Ice Cream Sandwich	1	3	3	2
Sherbet, all flavors	½ cup	3	3	1
Ice cream, rich (high fat)	½ cup	6	4	7
FRUIT SPREADS & SWEET TOPPINGS				
Syrup, light	2 tbsp	2	1	0
Chocolate syrup	1 tbsp	1	2	0
Cranberry sauce, jellied	1 tbsp	1	2	0
Honey	1 tbsp	2	2	0
Jam, Jelly or Preserves	1 tbsp	1	2	0
Syrup, regular	1 tbsp	2	2	0
Apple Butter	1 tbsp	2	3	0
FRUITS				
CANNED				
Applesauce, unsweetened	½ cup	1	2	0
Apricots	½ cup	1	2	0
Cherries	½ cup	1	2	0
Fruit cocktail	½ cup	1	2	0
Mandarin Oranges, drained	¾ cup	1	2	0
Peaches	½ cup	1	2	0
Pears	½ cup	1	2	0
Pineapple	½ cup	1	2	0
Plums	½ cup	1	2	0
DRIED				
Apples	4 rings	1	2	0
Apricots	8 halves	1	2	0
Banana Chips	¼ cup	1	2	8
Coconut, sweetened	¼ cup	1	2	8
Dates	3	1	2	0
Figs	2	2	2	0
Prunes	3	1	2	0
Raisins	2 tbsp	1	2	0
FRESH				
Apple, small	1	1	2	0
Apricots	4	1	2	0
Berries (blackberries, blueberries)	¾ cup	1	2	0
Cantaloupe, cubed	1 cup	1	2	0
Cherries	12	1	2	0
Figs, medium	2	1	2	0
Grapefruit	½	1	2	0
Grapes	17	1	2	0
Honeydew, cubed	1 cup	1	2	0
Mango	½	1	2	0
Nectarine, small	1	1	2	0
Orange, small	1	1	2	0

LEAST TO MOST CARBOHYDRATES Food	Amt	Calories DOWN	Carbs ACROSS	Fat ACROSS
FRUITS (cont.)				
FRESH (cont.)				
Peaches, medium	1	1	2	0
Pears, small	1	1	2	0
Pineapple	¾ cup	1	2	0
Plums, small	2	1	2	0
Raspberries	1 cup	1	2	0
Strawberries	1¼ cup	1	2	0
Watermelon, cubed	1¼ cup	1	2	0
Banana, medium	1	2	3	0
GRAINS (cooked unless otherwise stated)				
Asian noodles	½ cup	2	2	0
Buckwheat	½ cup	2	2	0
Bulgur	½ cup	2	2	0
Couscous	½ cup	2	2	0
Pasta - macaroni, spaghetti, linguini, fettuccine, penne, etc.	½ cup	2	2	0
Potato Gnocchi	½ cup	3	2	3
Ramen Noodles	½ cup	2	2	2
Grits	½ cup	2	3	0
Millet	½ cup	3	3	0
Pearled Barley	½ cup	2	3	0
Rice- brown or white	½ cup	3	3	0
Cornmeal (dry)	¼ cup	3	4	1
Flour (dry)	¼ cup	3	4	0
GRAIN DISHES				
Rice Pilaf	½ cup	3	3	1
Spanish Rice	½ cup	2	3	1
LAMB (cooked without added fat unless noted)				
Ground	3 oz	5	0	7
Leg	3 oz	5	0	7
Loin	3 oz	5	0	6
Shoulder	3 oz	5	0	6
MAIN DISHES				
BEEF				
Meat Loaf	3 oz	4	1	4
Salisbury Steak	3 oz	4	1	5
Stew with Potatoes, Carrots, Peas and Gravy	1 cup	3	2	1
Chili Con Carne with Beans	1 cup	6	3	5
Corned Beef Hash	1 cup	8	3	10
Beef with Noodles in Tomato Sauce	1 cup	6	3	3
Stroganoff with Noodles	1 cup	8	4	8
Swedish Meatballs	1 cup	9	4	9
Pot Pie	1 cup	11	5	13

LEAST TO MOST CARBOHYDRATES Food	Amt	Calories DOWN	Carbs ACROSS	Fat ACROSS
MAIN DISHES (cont.)				
CHICKEN				
Chicken a la King	¾ cup	4	1	2
Fricassee	1 cup	6	1	7
Fried Steak	3 oz	5	1	7
With Barbecue Sauce	5 cups	5	1	5
With Dumplings	1 cup	7	3	7
With Noodles	1 cup	5	3	2
Pot Pie	1 cup	11	5	12
CHINESE				
Pork Egg Foo Yung	1	2	0	3
Stir Fried Pork and Vegetables	1 cup	7	0	4
Chicken and Vegetable Combo	1 cup	6	1	7
Chicken Chow Mein	1 cup	5	1	5
Kung Pao Chicken	1 cup	9	1	12
Moo Goo Gai Pan	1 cup	5	1	7
Sweet and Sour Pork	1 cup	5	1	10
Beef or Pork Egg Roll	2	5	2	5
Cashew Chicken	1 cup	13	2	18
Chop Suey with Beef and Pork	1 cup	6	2	7
Dim Sum with Pork	5	5	2	5
General Tso Chicken	1 cup	6	2	7
Fried Rice with Meat or Poultry	1 cup	7	5	5
ITALIAN				
Chicken or Turkey Cacciatore	5 oz	5	1	6
Veal Parmigiana	3 oz	4	1	5
Chicken or Turkey Tetrazzini	1 cup	7	3	8
Lasagna with Ground Beef	1 cup	6	3	6
Macaroni and Cheese	2/3 cup	7	3	8
Spaghetti and Meat Balls with Tomato Sauce	1 cup	7	5	5
JAPANESE				
Chicken Teriyaki	1 cup	7	2	3
Sushi with Vegetables and Fish	6 pc	4	5	0
MEXICAN				
Chicken Fajita	1	4	1	1
Beef and Cheese Quesadilla	1	4	2	4
Cheese Quesadilla	1	4	2	4
Bean and Cheese Burrito	1	2	3	2
Bean Burrito	1	7	3	6
Beef Burrito	1	7	3	8
Beef Taco or Tostada with Cheese, Lettuce, Tomato and Salsa	2	7	3	7
Cheese Enchilada	1	6	3	7
Bean Taco or Tostada with Cheese, Lettuce, Tomato, Salsa	2	7	5	6

LEAST TO MOST CARBOHYDRATES Food	Amt	Calories DOWN	Carbs ACROSS	Fat ACROSS
MAIN DISHES (cont.)				
MEXICAN (cont.)				
Pork Tamales	1	4	1	5
Chicken Taco	1	3	2	7
Nachos with Beans and Cheese	1 cup	5	2	5
Refried Bean and Cheese Burrito, 6-inch Tortilla	1	7	4	6
OTHER				
Lamb Stew	1 cup	5	2	2
Cheese Blintzes	2	5	3	5
Cheese Knish	2	8	4	9
Pierogi with Potato and Cheese	3	4	4	2
Corndog	1	9	7	7
PIZZA				
Cheese	1 slice	6	4	6
Hawaiian	1 slice	7	4	6
Pepperoni	1 slice	7	5	5
Cheese, thick crust	1 slice	8	7	6
SEAFOOD				
Crab Cakes	1	2	0	2
Fish Fillets, baked	3 oz	2	0	0
Baked Salmon with Cucumber Dill Sauce	1 serv	5	1	3
Bouillabaisse	1 cup	5	1	3
Japanese Fish Cake Tempura	3 oz	3	1	2
Shrimp, Breaded, Fried	3 oz	4	1	4
Fish Fillet, Batter Coated or Breaded, Fried	3 oz	4	2	4
Oysters Rockefeller	1 cup	6	3	7
Paella (Paella a la Marinera)	1 cup	7	3	4
Tuna Noodle Casserole with Peas and Mushrooms	1 cup	7	4	5
NUTS AND SEEDS				
NUTS (DRY ROASTED)				
Pecans	¼ cup	4	0	8
Walnuts	¼ cup	4	0	8
Macadamia nuts	¼ cup	5	1	10
Nuts: almonds, cashews, hazelnuts, peanuts, pistachios	¼ cup	4	1	7
NUT BUTTERS				
Almond, Cashew, Peanut Butter, Sesame	2 tbsp	4	1	7
Tahini Butter	2 tbsp	4	1	6
SEEDS (DRY ROASTED)				
Sesame Seeds	2 tsp	1	0	1
Flax Seed	3 tbsp	4	1	5
Sunflower Seed Kernels	¼ cup	4	1	6

LEAST TO MOST CARBOHYDRATES Food	Amt	Calories DOWN	Carbs ACROSS	Fat ACROSS
PIES				
Custard	1/8 pie	5	4	5
Pumpkin	1/8 pie	5	4	4
Fruit, 2 crusts	1/8 pie	6	5	5
Lemon Meringue	1/8 pie	7	6	6
Pecan	1/8 pie	9	8	8
PORK (cooked without added fat unless noted)				
Bacon	2 slices	2	0	3
Bacon, Canadian style	2 oz	2	0	2
Boston Butt	3 oz	5	0	6
Chop, Center Loin	3 oz	3	0	3
Chop, Top Loin	3 oz	5	0	6
Cured Ham	3 oz	3	0	3
Cutlet	3 oz	5	0	6
Ground	3 oz	6	0	9
Picnic	3 oz	5	0	6
Sausage	3 oz	6	0	9
Shoulder	3 oz	5	0	6
Spareribs	3 oz	6	0	9
Tenderloin	3 oz	3	0	3
Chop, fried	3 oz	5	1	5
POULTRY (Chicken and Turkey) AND GAME (cooked without added fat unless noted)				
CHICKEN				
Breast with skin	3 oz	3	0	3
Breast, Fried	3 oz	4	0	3
Breast, skinless	3 oz	3	0	1
Leg with skin	3 oz	4	0	4
Leg, Fried	3 oz	4	0	5
Leg, skinless	3 oz	3	0	3
Thigh with skin	3 oz	5	0	5
Thigh, Fried	3 oz	4	0	5
Thigh, skinless	3 oz	4	0	4
Wing, Fried	3 oz	5	0	7
Wing	3 oz	5	0	6
TURKEY				
Breast with skin	3 oz	3	0	2
Dark Meat with skin	3 oz	4	0	4
Ground Turkey	3 oz	4	0	4
Leg with skin	3 oz	4	0	3
Light Meat with skin	3 oz	3	0	3
Light Meat, skinless	3 oz	3	0	1

LEAST TO MOST CARBOHYDRATES Food	Amt	Calories DOWN	Carbs ACROSS	Fat ACROSS
POULTRY (Chicken and Turkey) AND GAME (cont.)				
GAME				
Cornish Game Hen with skin	3 oz	5	0	6
Deer or Venison Chops	3 oz	4	0	3
Duck with skin	3 oz	6	0	9
Goose with skin	3 oz	5	0	7
Rabbit	3 oz	3	0	3
SALADS				
Chef Salad with Turkey, Ham and Cheese	¾ cup	3	0	3
Caesar Salad with Dressing	1 cup	3	1	5
Cobb Salad with Dressing	1 cup	4	1	6
Coleslaw	¾ cup	1	1	1
Carrot Raisin Salad	½ cup	4	2	6
Macaroni Salad	½ cup	4	2	4
Potato Salad	½ cup	4	2	5
Tabouli, Tabbouleh or Tabouli	1 cup	4	2	6
SANDWICHES				
Hot Dog on Bun	1	5	2	6
Bologna with Margarine	1	5	3	5
Chicken Salad Spread	1	7	3	6
Chili Hot Dog with Bun	1	7	3	8
Corned Beef	1	5	3	4
Egg Salad	1	6	3	5
Grilled Cheese	1	6	3	6
Pastrami	1	7	3	7
Tuna Salad	1	8	3	9
Bacon and Egg Croissant	1	8	4	10
Bacon, Lettuce and Tomato with Mayonnaise	1	7	4	7
Breaded Chicken Fillet with Lettuce, Tomato and Mayonnaise	1	9	4	10
Broiled Chicken Fillet on Whole Wheat Roll with Lettuce, Tomato and Mayonnaise	1	7	4	3
Ham and Cheese	1	7	4	6
Meatball and Spaghetti Sauce Submarine on Roll	1	9	4	8
Cheeseburger, 1/4 lb. with Mayonnaise and Tomatoes	1	14	5	16
Peanut Butter and Jelly	1	7	5	6
Roast Beef Submarine with Mayonnaise and Vegetables	1	8	5	5
Turkey Submarine with Cheese, Lettuce, Tomato and Mayonnaise	1	12	6	10

LEAST TO MOST CARBOHYDRATES Food	Amt	Calories DOWN	Carbs ACROSS	Fat ACROSS
SNACKS				
Corn Chips	1 oz	3	2	4
Popcorn, Popped in Oil	3 cups	3	2	4
Potato Chips, light	1 oz	3	2	2
Pretzel Sticks, Thin	10	2	2	0
Rice cakes	2	1	2	0
Taro Chips	1 oz	3	2	3
Tortilla Chips	1 oz	3	2	3
Tortilla Chips, light	1 oz	3	2	2
Trail Mix	¼ cup	3	2	4
Bagel Chips	½ cup	2	3	1
Popcorn, Air Popped	3 ¾ cup	2	3	0
Popcorn, Caramel	1 cup	3	3	2
Potato Chips, baked	1 oz	2	3	1
Pretzel, Whole Wheat	1 oz	2	3	0
Tortilla Chips, baked	1 oz	1	3	0
Pretzel, Soft	1	4	5	1
SOUPS				
Chicken Broth	1 cup	1	0	1
Beef or Chicken Noodle	1 cup	2	1	1
Bird's Nest with Chicken, Ham, Noodles	1 cup	2	1	1
Onion Soup	1 cup	1	1	1
Oyster Stew (made with milk)	1 cup	3	1	3
Vegetable Beef	1 cup	2	1	1
Black Bean	1 cup	2	2	1
Chunky Bean with Ham	1 cup	5	2	3
Chunky Chicken Noodle	1 cup	4	2	2
Chunky Minestrone	1 cup	3	2	1
Chunky Potato Ham Chowder	1 cup	4	2	5
Cream of Asparagus (made with Milk)	1 cup	3	2	3
Cream of Mushroom (made with milk)	1 cup	4	2	5
Cream of Potato (made with milk)	1 cup	3	2	2
Lentil and Ham	1 cup	3	2	1
Manhattan Clam Chowder	1 cup	3	2	1
Ramen Noodle	1 cup	3	2	3
Split Pea with Ham	1 cup	4	3	2
Tomato (made with milk)	1 cup	3	3	2
Green Pea Soup (made with milk)	1 cup	5	4	3

LEAST TO MOST CARBOHYDRATES **Food**	Amt	Calories DOWN	Carbs ACROSS	Fat ACROSS
SWEETENERS				
Powdered Sugar	3 tbsp	1	1	0
White Granulated Sugar	3 tbsp	1	1	0
Honey	1 tbsp	1	2	0
Molasses	1 tbsp	1	2	0
VEGETABLES – Non-Starchy				
Generally, ½ cup cooked or 1 cup raw equals one serving. If DOWN is "0" and you eat two servings, count DOWN as 1 Dot				
Asparagus, cooked	½ cup	0	0	0
Bell or Sweet Pepper, cooked	½ cup	0	0	0
Cabbage (cooked): Green, Napa, Red, Savoy	½ cup	0	0	0
Cauliflower, cooked	½ cup	0	0	0
Celery Stalk	2	0	0	0
Cucumber, sliced	¾ cup	0	0	0
Greens (cooked): Beet, Collards, Kale, Mustard, Spinach, Swiss Chard	½ cup	0	0	0
Mushrooms, cooked	½ cup	0	0	0
Salad Greens: Butterhead, Boston, Bibb, Endive, Escarole, Iceberg, Spinach	1½ cups	0	0	0
Watercress	1 cup	0	0	0
Zucchini Summer Squash, cooked	½ cup	0	0	0
Artichoke Hearts, cooked	½ cup	1	1	0
Beans: Yellow, Green, String or Wax, cooked	2/3 cup	1	1	0
Beets, sliced, Canned	½ cup	1	1	0
Broccoli Spears, cooked	½ cup	1	1	0
Brussels Sprouts, cooked	½ cup	1	1	0
Carrots, cooked	2/3 cup	1	1	0
Eggplant, cooked	1 cup	1	1	0
Leeks, cooked	¾ cup	0	1	0
Onions, Chopped	¾ cup	0	1	0
Snow or Sugar Peas, cooked	½ cup	1	1	0
Tomato	1	1	1	0
Tomato Puree, Canned	¼ cup	1	1	0
VEGETABLE DISHES				
Vegetable Tempura	12 pc	3	2	5
Onion Rings, Breaded and Pan Fried	11	6	4	8

Food List: Least to Most Fat

LEAST TO MOST FAT Food	Amt	Calories DOWN	Carbs ACROSS	Fat ACROSS
BEEF (cooked without fat)				
Eye of Round	3 oz	3	0	2
Veal (ground)	3 oz	3	0	2
Bottom Round	3 oz	4	0	3
Round	3 oz	4	0	3
Round Tip	3 oz	4	0	3
Top Round	3 oz	4	0	3
Veal Shoulder, Arm	3 oz	3	0	3
Flank Steak	3 oz	4	0	4
Top Sirloin	3 oz	4	0	4
Veal Loin	3 oz	4	0	4
Ground Beef, extra lean	3 oz	3	0	5
Top Loin	3 oz	4	0	5
Ground Beef, lean	3 oz	5	0	6
T-Bone	3 oz	5	0	6
Tenderloin	3 oz	5	0	6
Ground Beef, regular	3 oz	5	0	7
Porterhouse	3 oz	5	0	7
Rib Eye	3 oz	5	0	7
Short Ribs	3 oz	5	0	7
Ribs	3 oz	6	0	8
BEVERAGES				
ALCOHOL				
Beer	12 fl oz	3	2	0
Distilled spirits (gin, rum, vodka, whiskey, Scotch)	1 fl oz	1	0	0
Liqueurs	1 fl oz	2	2	0
Port	4 fl oz	3	1	0
Red or white wine	4 fl oz	2	0	0
Sherry, Dry	4 fl oz	3	1	0
ESPRESSO (Get Nutrition Facts at coffee shop and convert to dots)				
Tall Latte w/ Nonfat Milk	12 fl oz	2	2	0
Tall Mocha w/ Whole Milk	12 fl oz	4	3	3
Tall Latte w/ Whole Milk	12 fl oz	4	2	4
JUICE and NECTARS				
Apple	8 fl oz	2	3	0
Apricot	8 fl oz	3	4	0
Carrot	8 fl oz	2	3	0
Cranberry Cocktail	8 fl oz	3	4	0
Fruit Punch Drink	8 fl oz	2	4	0
Grape	8 fl oz	3	4	0
Grapefruit	8 fl oz	2	3	0
Lemonade	8 fl oz	2	3	0
Orange	8 fl oz	2	3	0
Papaya	8 fl oz	3	4	0

LEAST TO MOST FAT Food	Amt	Calories DOWN	Carbs ACROSS	Fat ACROSS
BEVERAGES (cont.)				
JUICE and NECTARS (cont.)				
Peach	8 fl oz	3	4	0
Pear	8 fl oz	3	5	0
Prune	8 fl oz	4	5	0
Tomato	8 fl oz	1	1	0
OTHER				
Cocoa	8 fl oz	3	3	0
Hot Cider	8 fl oz	2	3	0
Soda	8 fl oz	2	3	0
Milkshake, Vanilla	8 fl oz	5	5	3
Eggnog	8 fl oz	7	4	7
BREADS				
BAGELS				
All flavors (small)	1	4	5	0
Whole wheat; whole grain (small)	1	4	4	0
BISCUITS, ROLLS, ETC.				
Baking Powder, Buttermilk	1	3	3	3
Bun — Hot dog or Hamburger	1	3	4	0
Corn Pone, Baked	1	3	3	1
Cornbread (2½" square)	1 pc	3	3	1
Crumpet	1	2	2	0
English muffin	1	3	4	0
Roll — Egg dinner	1	2	2	1
Roll — Hawaiian Sweet Bread	1	2	2	1
Roll — Plain (small)	1	2	2	0
Scone	1	3	2	2
OTHER				
Bread sticks (4" x ½")	4	2	2	0
Pita (6" across)	1	3	4	0
Seasoned Croutons, Ready to Eat	¼ cup	1	1	1
Taco Shells	2	2	2	2
Tortilla, corn (6" across)	1	2	2	0
Tortilla, flour (6" across)	1	2	2	0
SLICED BREAD				
Cinnamon, potato, rye, sourdough, white	1 slice	2	2	0
Whole-wheat, whole grain	1 slice	2	1	0
CAKES				
Angel Food Cake (1/12 of cake)	1 slice	3	4	0
Cake without frosting (2½" square)	1 pc	4	4	2
Fruitcake (1" slice)	1 pc	3	3	2
Brownie (2" square)	1 pc	3	3	3
Fruit Fritter	1	4	3	3
Brownie with Chocolate Icing (2" square)	1 pc	4	4	4
Cake with frosting (2½" square)	1 pc	5	4	4

LEAST TO MOST FAT Food	Amt	Calories DOWN	Carbs ACROSS	Fat ACROSS
CAKES (cont.)				
Cupcake with frosting (small)	1	5	4	4
Pineapple Upside Down Cake (2" square)	1 pc	5	4	4
Carrot Cake (3" square)	1 pc	5	4	5
Doughnut, Glazed	1	5	3	5
Doughnut, Plain Old Fashioned	1	4	3	5
Pound Cake (1½" slice)	1 pc	6	5	5
Doughnut with Creme Filling	1	6	3	6
Doughnut with Jelly Filling	1	6	4	6
Cheesecake (1/12 of cake)	1 slice	4	4	10
CANDY				
Fruit Leather Bar or Roll	1	2	2	0
Hard Candy	2	1	1	0
Jelly Beans	15	3	5	0
Marshmallows	4	2	3	0
Chocolate Fudge	1 oz	3	3	1
Peanut Brittle	1½ oz	4	4	1
Chocolate Chip Granola Bar	1	4	3	2
Almond Paste	2 tbsp	3	2	3
Semi Sweet or Milk Choc Chips	1 oz	3	2	3
Chocolate Bar with Almonds	3 oz	5	3	5
Milk Chocolate Bar	3¼ oz	5	3	5
CEREALS				
Cereals, cooked	½ cup	2	2	0
Cereals, sweetened, ready-to-eat	½ cup	2	2	0
Cereals, unsweetened, ready-to-eat	¾ cup	2	2	0
Corn Grits, cooked	½ cup	1	2	0
Puffed Cereal	1½ cups	2	2	0
Granola, low-fat	¼ cup	2	2	1
Granola	¼ cup	3	1	3
CHEESE				
Cottage Cheese, Low Fat 1%	½ cup	2	0	0
Cream Cheese, Fat Free	2 tbsp	1	0	0
Cottage Cheese, Low Fat 2%	½ cup	2	0	1
Parmesan or Romano Cheese, Grated	2 tbsp	1	0	1
Feta Cheese	1 oz	1	0	2
Mozzarella Cheese, Part Skim Milk, Low Moisture	1 oz	2	0	2
Ricotta Cheese, Part Skim Milk	¼ cup	2	0	2
American Cheese, Processed	1 oz	2	0	3
Blue Cheese	1 oz	2	0	3
Brie Cheese	1 oz	2	0	3
Cream Cheese, Light	1 oz	1	0	3
Gouda Cheese	1 oz	2	0	3
Gruyere Cheese	1 oz	2	0	3
Monterey Jack Cheese	1 oz	2	0	3

LEAST TO MOST FAT Food	Amt	Calories DOWN	Carbs ACROSS	Fat ACROSS
CHEESE (cont.)				
Provolone Cheese	1 oz	2	0	3
Swiss Cheese	1 oz	2	0	3
Cheddar Cheese	1 oz	2	0	4
Cream Cheese	2 tbsp	2	0	4
COBBLERS & CRISPS				
Fruit Cobbler	1 serv	4	5	2
Fruit Crisp	½ cup	5	6	3
COFFEE CAKES, MUFFINS, QUICK BREADS, PANCAKES, & WAFFLES				
Muffin, cake (small)	1	3	3	2
Toaster Pastry, fruit	1	4	4	2
Waffle, plain (frozen)	2	4	4	2
Cinnamon Bun, frosted	1	4	4	3
Coffeecake — cheese, fruit, cinnamon (2½" slice)	1 pc	4	4	3
Quick Breads (banana, zucchini, nuts; 1½" slice)	1 pc	3	2	3
French Toast, baked	2 slices	7	5	4
Pancakes, plain	3	5	4	4
Danish Pastry, plain	1	4	3	5
CONDIMENTS & SAUCES				
Barbecue Sauce	2 tbsp	1	1	0
Catsup or Ketchup	2 tbsp	1	1	0
Chutney	1 tbsp	1	1	0
Cocktail Sauce	¼ cup	1	2	0
Hot Dog Pickle Relish	2 tbsp	1	1	0
Mustard	1 tbsp	0	0	0
Plum Sauce	1 tbsp	1	1	0
Mayonnaise, Low calorie	1 tbsp	1	0	1
Olives - large	8 items	1	0	1
Tartar Sauce	2 tbsp	2	0	1
Guacamole	2 tbsp	1	0	2
Mayonnaise	1 tbsp	2	0	3
COOKIES				
Fortune cookie	4	2	3	0
Fig Bar	2	2	3	1
Gingersnaps	2	1	1	1
Puffed Rice Cereal and Marshmallow (2" square)	1	2	3	1
Animal Crackers	12	3	3	2
Butter cookie	6	3	2	2
Chocolate or Vanilla Wafer	5	3	3	2
Sugar cookie (2" across)	2	3	2	2
Vanilla or Chocolate Sandwich with Creme Filling	3	3	2	2
Chocolate Chip (1½" across)	1	3	2	3
Oatmeal cookie	1	4	3	3
Shortbread cookie	4	3	2	3

LEAST TO MOST FAT Food	Amt	Calories DOWN	Carbs ACROSS	Fat ACROSS
CRACKERS				
Matzo Crackers	1	2	3	0
Melba Toast	3	1	1	0
Rye Crispbread Crackers	1	1	1	0
Graham Crackers (2½" sq)	4	2	3	1
Oyster crackers	20	1	1	1
Saltine Crackers	5	1	1	1
Whole Wheat Crackers	7	2	2	2
Cheese Cracker Sandwich with Peanut Butter	4	3	2	3
Cheese Crackers	30	3	2	3
CRUSTS				
Pizza Crust	1/8 pie	3	3	1
Graham Cracker Pie Crust	1/8 pie	3	2	3
Pie Crust, Baked	1/8 pie	2	1	3
Vanilla Wafer Pie Crust	1/8 pie	2	1	3
CUSTARD & PUDDINGS				
Pudding, sugar-free (made with 2% milk)	½ cup	2	1	1
Reduced Calorie Gelatin Mix with Aspartame	½ cup	1	1	0
Gelatin, regular	½ cup	2	2	0
Egg Custard (made with 2% milk)	½ cup	3	3	1
Pudding, regular (made with 2% milk)	½ cup	3	3	1
Rice Pudding	½ cup	4	3	2
DAIRY				
CREAM				
Creamer, Non-Dairy, Lite, liquid	2 tbsp	0	0	0
Substitute, Powder	1 tsp	0	0	0
Creamer, Non-Dairy, liquid	2 tbsp	1	0	1
Half and Half	2 tbsp	1	0	1
Heavy, Whipped	2 tbsp	1	0	2
Whipping, Heavy, Liquid	2 tbsp	2	0	4
Whipping, Light, Liquid	2 tbsp	2	0	4
MILK				
Nonfat, skim	1 cup	2	1	0
1% Low-fat	1 cup	2	1	1
Condensed, sweetened	2 tbsp	2	2	1
Evaporated, whole	2 tbsp	1	0	1
2% Reduced Fat	1 cup	2	1	2
Soy	1 cup	2	1	2
3.3% Whole	1 cup	3	1	3

LEAST TO MOST FAT Food	Amt	Calories DOWN	Carbs ACROSS	Fat ACROSS
DAIRY (cont.)				
SOUR CREAM				
Fat Free	2 tbsp	0	1	0
Reduced Fat	2 tbsp	1	0	1
Regular	2 tbsp	1	0	2
YOGURT				
Fruit, Non-Fat, Sweetened with Low Calorie Sweetener	1 cup	2	2	0
Plain, Non-Fat	1 cup	3	2	0
Fruit, Low Fat	1 cup	5	6	1
Plain, Whole Milk	1 cup	3	1	3
EGGS AND EGG DISHES				
Egg White, Raw	1	0	0	0
Egg Substitute, Liquid	¼ cup	1	0	1
Egg, Raw	1	1	0	2
Egg Omelet	1	2	0	3
Scrambled Eggs	¼ cup	2	0	3
Western Omelet with Ham, Onions and Peppers	1	2	0	3
Cheese Omelet	1	3	0	4
Egg Yolk, Raw	3	4	0	6
Eggs Benedict	1	6	2	7
FAST-FOOD				
BREAKFASTS				
Bacon, Egg & Cheese Biscuit	1	9	4	9
Sausage Biscuit with Egg	1	10	4	12
FRENCH FRIES				
Small French Fries	1 order	5	4	4
Medium French Fries	1 order	7	6	6
Large French Fries	1 order	10	8	10
SALADS				
Caesar Salad (without chicken)	1 order	2	1	2
Caesar Salad with Grilled Chicken	1 order	4	1	2
Caesar Salad with Crispy Chicken	1 order	6	3	5
SANDWICHES AND ENTREES				
Hamburger	1	5	4	3
Cheeseburger	1	6	4	5
Fish Filets	1	8	5	7
Crispy Chicken Pieces	1	10	6	9
Double Cheeseburger	1	9	4	9

LEAST TO MOST FAT Food	Amt	Calories DOWN	Carbs ACROSS	Fat ACROSS
FAST-FOOD (cont.)				
SHAKES				
Shake (small)	12 fl oz	9	9	4
Shake (medium)	16 fl oz	12	12	5
Shake (large)	21 fl oz	15	16	7
FATS				
Salad Dressing: Italian	2 tbsp	2	0	3
Avocado	½ cup	2	1	4
Butter, whipped	1 tbsp	2	0	4
Margarine	1 tbsp	2	0	4
Salad Dressing: Thousand Island	2 tbsp	2	1	4
Butter	1 tbsp	2	0	5
Chicken Fat	1 tbsp	2	0	5
Lard	1 tbsp	2	0	5
Oil: almond. canola, coconut, corn, hazelnut, olive, peanut, safflower, sesame, soybean, sunflower, walnut	1 tbsp	2	0	5
Shortening	1 tbsp	2	0	5
FISN AND SHELLFISH (Unless noted, cooked without added fat)				
FIN FISH				
Cod	3 oz	2	0	0
Lingcod	3 oz	2	0	0
Mahi Mahi, Dolphinfish or Dorado	3 oz	2	0	0
Pollock	3 oz	2	0	0
Surimi	3 oz	2	1	0
Tuna, Canned in Water, Drained	2 oz	1	0	0
Yellowfin Tuna	3 oz	2	0	0
Tuna, Canned in Water, Drained	2 oz	1	0	0
Yellowfin Tuna	3 oz	2	0	0
Gefilte Fish, Sweet Recipe	3 oz	1	1	1
Halibut	3 oz	2	0	1
Monkfish	3 oz	2	0	1
Freshwater Bass	3 oz	2	0	2
Rainbow Trout, Farmed	3 oz	3	0	2
Swordfish	2 oz	3	0	2
Whitefish	3 oz	3	0	2
Swordfish	2 oz	3	0	2
Whitefish	3 oz	3	0	2
Butterfish	3 oz	3	0	3
Catfish	3 oz	3	0	3
Pompano	3 oz	4	0	4
Salmon	3 oz	4	0	4
Eel	3 oz	4	0	5

LEAST TO MOST FAT **Food**	**Amt**	**Calories DOWN**	**Carbs ACROSS**	**Fat ACROSS**
FISN AND SHELLFISH (cont.)				
SEAFOOD				
Crayfish	3 oz	1	0	0
Dungeness Crab	3 oz	2	0	0
Northern Lobster	3 oz	2	0	0
Shrimp	3 oz	2	0	0
Alaska King Crab	3 oz	2	0	1
Blue Mussel	3 oz	3	0	1
Clams	3 oz	3	0	1
Eastern Oyster	3 oz	1	0	1
Scallops	3 oz	2	0	1
Oysters	3 oz	2	0	2
FRANKS, SAUSAGES, JERKY AND LUNCHEON MEATS				
FRANKS AND SAUSAGES				
Frankfurter, Chicken	2 oz	2	0	3
Frankfurter, Turkey	2 oz	2	0	3
Frankfurter, Beef	2 oz	3	0	5
Beef and Pork Frankfurter	2 oz	4	0	6
Beef and Pork Knockwurst	2 oz	3	0	6
Pork Bratwurst	2 oz	3	0	6
Pork Sausage Link	2 oz	4	0	7
Beef and Pork Chorizo	2 oz	5	0	8
Beef and Pork Pepperoni	2 oz	6	0	10
JERKY				
Pork Jerky	1 oz	2	0	2
Beef Jerky	1 oz	2	0	3
LUNCHEON MEAT				
Roast beef	2 oz	1	0	0
Turkey breast	1 oz	1	0	0
Corned beef	2 oz	1	0	1
Ham, turkey	2 oz	1	0	1
Pastrami, turkey	2 oz	2	0	1
Ham	2 oz	2	0	2
Prosciutto Ham	2 oz	2	0	2
Bologna, turkey	1 oz	2	0	3
Salami, turkey	2 oz	2	0	3
Salami, beef	2 oz	3	0	4
Bologna, beef	2 oz	4	0	6
FROZEN DESSERTS				
Popsicle	1	1	1	0
Ice cream, light	½ cup	2	2	1
Sherbet, all flavors	½ cup	3	3	1
Frozen Yogurt, fruit varieties	½ cup	3	3	2
Frozen Yogurt, Vanilla (soft)	½ cup	2	2	2
Ice Cream Sandwich	1	3	3	2

LEAST TO MOST FAT Food	Amt	Calories DOWN	Carbs ACROSS	Fat ACROSS
FROZEN DESSERTS (cont.)				
Choc Covered Ice Cream Bar	1	3	2	5
Ice cream, regular	½ cup	3	2	3
Ice cream, rich (high fat)	½ cup	6	4	7
FRUIT SPREADS & SWEET TOPPINGS				
Apple Butter	1 tbsp	2	3	0
Chocolate syrup	1 tbsp	1	2	0
Cranberry sauce, jellied	1 tbsp	1	2	0
Honey	1 tbsp	2	2	0
Jam, Jelly or Preserves	1 tbsp	1	2	0
Syrup, light	2 tbsp	2	1	0
Syrup, regular	1 tbsp	2	2	0
FRUITS				
CANNED				
Applesauce, unsweetened	½ cup	1	2	0
Apricots	½ cup	1	2	0
Cherries	½ cup	1	2	0
Fruit cocktail	½ cup	1	2	0
Mandarin Oranges, drained	¾ cup	1	2	0
Peaches	½ cup	1	2	0
Pears	½ cup	1	2	0
Pineapple	½ cup	1	2	0
Plums	½ cup	1	2	0
DRIED				
Apples	4 rings	1	2	0
Apricots	8 halves	1	2	0
Dates	3	1	2	0
Figs	2	2	2	0
Prunes	3	1	2	0
Raisins	2 tbsp	1	2	0
Banana Chips	¼ cup	1	2	8
Coconut, sweetened	¼ cup	1	2	8
FRESH				
Apple, small	1	1	2	0
Apricots	4	1	2	0
Banana, medium	1	2	3	0
Berries (blackberries, blueberries)	¾ cup	1	2	0
Cantaloupe, cubed	1 cup	1	2	0
Cherries	12	1	2	0
Figs, medium	2	1	2	0
Grapefruit	½	1	2	0
Grapes	17	1	2	0
Honeydew, cubed	1 cup	1	2	0
Mango	½	1	2	0
Nectarine, small	1	1	2	0

LEAST TO MOST FAT Food	Amt	Calories DOWN	Carbs ACROSS	Fat ACROSS
FRUITS (cont.)				
FRESH (cont.)				
Orange, small	1	1	2	0
Peaches, medium	1	1	2	0
Pears, small	1	1	2	0
Pineapple	¾ cup	1	2	0
Plums, small	2	1	2	0
Raspberries	1 cup	1	2	0
Strawberries	1¼ cup	1	2	0
Watermelon, cubed	1¼ cup	1	2	0
GRAINS (cooked unless otherwise stated)				
Asian noodles	½ cup	2	2	0
Buckwheat	½ cup	2	2	0
Bulgur	½ cup	2	2	0
Couscous	½ cup	2	2	0
Flour (dry)	¼ cup	3	4	0
Grits	½ cup	2	3	0
Millet	½ cup	3	3	0
Pasta - macaroni, spaghetti, linguini, fettuccine, penne, etc.	½ cup	2	2	0
Pearled Barley	½ cup	2	3	0
Rice- brown or white	½ cup	3	3	0
Cornmeal (dry)	¼ cup	3	4	1
Ramen Noodles	½ cup	2	2	2
Potato Gnocchi	½ cup	3	2	3
GRAIN DISHES				
Rice Pilaf	½ cup	3	3	1
Spanish Rice	½ cup	2	3	1
LAMB (cooked without added fat unless noted)				
Loin	3 oz	5	0	6
Shoulder	3 oz	5	0	6
Ground	3 oz	5	0	7
Leg	3 oz	5	0	7
MAIN DISHES				
BEEF				
Stew with Potatoes, Carrots, Peas and Gravy	1 cup	3	2	1
Beef with Noodles in Tomato Sauce	1 cup	6	3	3
Meat Loaf	3 oz	4	1	4
Chili Con Carne with Beans	1 cup	6	3	5
Salisbury Steak	3 oz	4	1	5
Stroganoff with Noodles	1 cup	8	4	8
Swedish Meatballs	1 cup	9	4	9
Corned Beef Hash	1 cup	8	3	10
Pot Pie	1 cup	11	5	13

LEAST TO MOST FAT Food	Amt	Calories DOWN	Carbs ACROSS	Fat ACROSS
MAIN DISHES (cont.)				
CHICKEN				
Chicken a la King	¾ cup	4	1	2
With Noodles	1 cup	5	3	2
With Barbecue Sauce	5 cups	5	1	5
Fricassee	1 cup	6	1	7
Fried Steak	3 oz	5	1	7
With Dumplings	1 cup	7	3	7
Pot Pie	1 cup	11	5	12
CHINESE				
Pork Egg Foo Yung	1	2	0	3
Sweet and Sour Pork	1 cup	5	3	3
Stir Fried Pork and Vegetables	1 cup	7	0	4
Kung Pao Chicken	1 cup	4	1	4
Beef or Pork Egg Roll	2	5	2	5
Chicken Chow Mein	1 cup	5	1	5
Dim Sum with Pork	5	5	2	5
Fried Rice with Meat or Poultry	1 cup	7	5	5
Chicken and Vegetable Combo	1 cup	6	1	7
Chop Suey with Beef and Pork	1 cup	6	2	7
General Tso Chicken	1 cup	6	2	7
Moo Goo Gai Pan	1 cup	5	1	7
Cashew Chicken	1 cup	6	2	7
ITALIAN				
Spaghetti and Meat Balls with Tomato Sauce	1 cup	7	5	5
Veal Parmigiana	3 oz	4	1	5
Chicken or Turkey Cacciatore	5 oz	5	1	6
Lasagna with Ground Beef	1 cup	6	3	6
Chicken or Turkey Tetrazzini	1 cup	7	3	8
Macaroni and Cheese	2/3 cup	7	3	8
JAPANESE				
Sushi with Vegetables and Fish	6 pc	4	5	0
Chicken Teriyaki	1 cup	7	2	3
MEXICAN				
Chicken Fajita	1	4	1	1
Bean and Cheese Burrito	1	2	3	2
Beef and Cheese Quesadilla	1	4	2	4
Cheese Quesadilla	1	4	2	4
Nachos with Beans and Cheese	1 cup	5	2	5
Pork Tamales	1	4	1	5
Bean Burrito	1	7	3	6
Bean Taco or Tostada with Cheese, Lettuce, Tomato, Salsa	2	7	5	6
Refried Bean and Cheese Burrito, 6-inch Tortilla	1	7	4	6
Beef Taco or Tostada with Cheese, Lettuce, Tomato and Salsa	2	7	3	7

LEAST TO MOST FAT Food	Amt	Calories DOWN	Carbs ACROSS	Fat ACROSS
MAIN DISHES (cont.)				
MEXICAN (cont.)				
Cheese Enchilada	1	6	3	7
Chicken Taco	1	3	2	7
Beef Burrito	1	7	3	8
OTHER				
Lamb Stew	1 cup	5	2	2
Pierogi with Potato and Cheese	3	4	4	2
Cheese Blintzes	2	5	3	5
Corndog	1	9	7	7
Cheese Knish	2	8	4	9
PIZZA				
Pepperoni	1 slice	7	5	5
Cheese	1 slice	6	4	6
Cheese, thick crust	1 slice	8	7	6
Hawaiian	1 slice	7	4	6
SEAFOOD				
Fish Fillets, baked	3 oz	2	0	0
Crab Cakes	1	2	0	2
Japanese Fish Cake Tempura	3 oz	3	1	2
Baked Salmon with Cucumber Dill Sauce	1 serv	5	1	3
Bouillabaisse	1 cup	5	1	3
Fish Fillet, Batter Coated or Breaded, Fried	3 oz	4	2	4
Paella (Paella a la Marinera)	1 cup	7	3	4
Shrimp, Breaded, Fried	3 oz	4	1	4
Tuna Noodle Casserole with Peas and Mushrooms	1 cup	7	4	5
Oysters Rockefeller	1 cup	6	3	7
NUTS AND SEEDS				
NUTS (DRY ROASTED)				
Nuts: almonds, cashews, hazelnuts, peanuts, pistachios	¼ cup	4	1	7
Pecans	¼ cup	4	0	8
Walnuts	¼ cup	4	0	8
Macadamia nuts	¼ cup	5	1	10
NUT BUTTERS				
Tahini Butter	2 tbsp	4	1	6
Almond, Cashew, Peanut Butter, Sesame	2 tbsp	4	1	7
SEEDS (DRY ROASTED)				
Sesame Seeds	2 tsp	1	0	1
Flax Seed	3 tbsp	4	1	5
Sunflower Seed Kernels	¼ cup	4	1	6

LEAST TO MOST FAT Food	Amt	Calories DOWN	Carbs ACROSS	Fat ACROSS
PIES				
Pumpkin	1/8 pie	5	4	4
Custard	1/8 pie	5	4	5
Fruit, 2 crusts	1/8 pie	6	5	5
Lemon Meringue	1/8 pie	7	6	6
Pecan	1/8 pie	9	8	8
PORK (cooked without added fat unless noted)				
Bacon, Canadian style	2 oz	2	0	2
Bacon	2 slices	2	0	3
Chop, Center Loin	3 oz	3	0	3
Cured Ham	3 oz	3	0	3
Tenderloin	3 oz	3	0	3
Chop, fried	3 oz	5	1	5
Boston Butt	3 oz	5	0	6
Chop, Top Loin	3 oz	5	0	6
Cutlet	3 oz	5	0	6
Picnic	3 oz	5	0	6
Shoulder	3 oz	5	0	6
Ground	3 oz	6	0	9
Sausage	3 oz	6	0	9
Spareribs	3 oz	6	0	9
POULTRY (Chicken and Turkey) AND GAME (cooked without added fat unless noted)				
CHICKEN				
Breast, skinless	3 oz	3	0	1
Breast with skin	3 oz	3	0	3
Breast, Fried	3 oz	4	0	3
Leg, skinless	3 oz	3	0	3
Leg with skin	3 oz	4	0	4
Thigh, skinless	3 oz	4	0	4
Leg, Fried	3 oz	4	0	5
Thigh with skin	3 oz	5	0	5
Thigh, Fried	3 oz	4	0	5
Wing	3 oz	5	0	6
Wing, Fried	3 oz	5	0	7
TURKEY				
Light Meat, skinless	3 oz	3	0	1
Breast with skin	3 oz	3	0	2
Leg with skin	3 oz	4	0	3
Light Meat with skin	3 oz	3	0	3
Dark Meat with skin	3 oz	4	0	4
Ground Turkey	3 oz	4	0	4

LEAST TO MOST FAT Food	Amt	Calories DOWN	Carbs ACROSS	Fat ACROSS
POULTRY (Chicken and Turkey) AND GAME (cont.)				
GAME				
Deer or Venison Chops	3 oz	4	0	3
Rabbit	3 oz	3	0	3
Cornish Game Hen with skin	3 oz	5	0	6
Goose with skin	3 oz	5	0	7
Duck with skin	3 oz	6	0	9
SALADS				
Coleslaw	¾ cup	1	1	1
Chef Salad with Turkey, Ham and Cheese	¾ cup	3	0	3
Macaroni Salad	½ cup	4	2	4
Caesar Salad with Dressing	1 cup	3	1	5
Potato Salad	½ cup	4	2	5
Carrot Raisin Salad	½ cup	4	2	6
Cobb Salad with Dressing	1 cup	4	1	6
Tabouli, Tabbouleh or Tabouli	1 cup	4	2	6
SANDWICHES				
Broiled Chicken Fillet on Whole Wheat Roll with Lettuce, Tomato and Mayonnaise	1	7	4	3
Turkey Submarine with Cheese, Lettuce, Tomato and Mayonnaise	1	5	5	3
Corned Beef	1	5	3	4
Bologna with Margarine	1	5	3	5
Egg Salad	1	6	3	5
Roast Beef Submarine with Mayonnaise and Vegetables	1	8	5	5
Chicken Salad Spread	1	7	3	6
Grilled Cheese	1	6	3	6
Ham and Cheese	1	7	4	6
Hot Dog on Bun	1	5	2	6
Peanut Butter and Jelly	1	7	5	6
Bacon, Lettuce and Tomato with Mayonnaise	1	7	4	7
Pastrami	1	7	3	7
Chili Hot Dog with Bun	1	7	3	8
Meatball and Spaghetti Sauce Submarine on Roll	1	9	4	8
Tuna Salad	1	8	3	9
Bacon and Egg Croissant	1	8	4	10
Breaded Chicken Fillet with Lettuce, Tomato and Mayonnaise	1	8	4	10
Cheeseburger, 1/4 lb. with Mayonnaise and Tomatoes	1	11	5	13

LEAST TO MOST FAT Food	Amt	Calories DOWN	Carbs ACROSS	Fat ACROSS
SNACKS				
Popcorn, Air Popped	3 ¾ cup	2	3	0
Pretzel Sticks, Thin	10	2	2	0
Pretzel, Whole Wheat	1 oz	2	3	0
Rice cakes	2	1	2	0
Tortilla Chips, baked	1 oz	1	3	0
Bagel Chips	½ cup	2	3	1
Potato Chips, baked	1 oz	2	3	1
Pretzel, Soft	1	4	5	1
Popcorn, Caramel	1 cup	3	3	2
Potato Chips, light	1 oz	3	2	2
Tortilla Chips, light	1 oz	3	2	2
Taro Chips	1 oz	3	2	3
Tortilla Chips	1 oz	3	2	3
Corn Chips	1 oz	3	2	4
Popcorn, Popped in Oil	3 cups	3	2	4
Trail Mix	¼ cup	3	2	4
SOUPS				
Beef or Chicken Noodle	1 cup	2	1	1
Bird's Nest with Chicken, Ham, Noodles	1 cup	2	1	1
Black Bean	1 cup	2	2	1
Chicken Broth	1 cup	1	0	1
Chunky Minestrone	1 cup	3	2	1
Lentil and Ham	1 cup	3	2	1
Manhattan Clam Chowder	1 cup	3	2	1
Onion Soup	1 cup	1	1	1
Vegetable Beef	1 cup	2	1	1
Chunky Chicken Noodle	1 cup	4	2	2
Cream of Potato (made with milk)	1 cup	3	2	2
Split Pea with Ham	1 cup	4	3	2
Tomato (made with milk)	1 cup	3	3	2
Chunky Bean with Ham	1 cup	5	2	3
Cream of Asparagus (made with Milk)	1 cup	3	2	3
Green Pea Soup (made with milk)	1 cup	5	4	3
Oyster Stew (made with milk)	1 cup	3	1	3
Ramen Noodle	1 cup	3	2	3
Chunky Potato Ham Chowder	1 cup	4	2	5
Cream of Mushroom (made with milk)	1 cup	4	2	5

LEAST TO MOST FAT Food	Amt	Calories DOWN	Carbs ACROSS	Fat ACROSS
SWEETENERS				
Honey	1 tbsp	1	2	0
Molasses	1 tbsp	1	2	0
Powdered Sugar	3 tbsp	1	1	0
White Granulated Sugar	3 tbsp	1	1	0
VEGETABLES – Non-Starchy				
Generally, ½ cup cooked or 1 cup raw equals one serving. If DOWN is "0" and you eat two servings, count DOWN as 1 Dot				
Artichoke Hearts, cooked	½ cup	1	1	0
Asparagus, cooked	½ cup	0	0	0
Beans: Yellow, Green, String or Wax, cooked	2/3 cup	1	1	0
Beets, sliced, Canned	½ cup	1	1	0
Bell or Sweet Pepper, cooked	½ cup	0	0	0
Broccoli Spears, cooked	½ cup	1	1	0
Brussels Sprouts, cooked	½ cup	1	1	0
Cabbage (cooked): Green, Napa, Red, Savoy	½ cup	0	0	0
Carrots, cooked	2/3 cup	1	1	0
Cauliflower, cooked	½ cup	0	0	0
Celery Stalk	2	0	0	0
Cucumber, sliced	¾ cup	0	0	0
Eggplant, cooked	1 cup	1	1	0
Greens (cooked): Beet, Collards, Kale, Mustard, Spinach, Swiss Chard	½ cup	0	0	0
Leeks, cooked	¾ cup	0	1	0
Mushrooms, cooked	½ cup	0	0	0
Onions, Chopped	¾ cup	0	1	0
Salad Greens: Butterhead, Boston, Bibb, Endive, Escarole, Iceberg, Spinach	1½ cups	0	0	0
Snow or Sugar Peas, cooked	½ cup	1	1	0
Tomato	1	1	1	0
Tomato Puree, Canned	¼ cup	1	1	0
Watercress	1 cup	0	0	0
Zucchini Summer Squash, cooked	½ cup	0	0	0
VEGETABLE DISHES				
Vegetable Tempura	12 pc	3	2	5
Onion Rings, Breaded and Pan Fried	11	6	4	8

LEAST TO MOST FAT Food	Amt	Calories DOWN	Carbs ACROSS	Fat ACROSS
VEGETABLES —Starchy				
BEANS				
Blackeye, garbanzo, kidney, lentils, lima, navy, pinto, Split pea	½ cup	2	1	0
Baked Beans	½ cup	4	3	1
Refried	½ cup	2	2	1
Soybeans, boiled	½ cup	3	0	3
CORN				
White Hominy	½ cup	1	1	0
White, Yellow, or Creamed	½ cup	2	3	0
GREEN PEAS				
Green Peas	½ cup	1	1	0
Green Peas and Carrots	½ cup	1	1	0
OTHER				
Jerusalem Artichoke	½ cup	1	2	0
Parsnips	½ cup	1	2	0
Pumpkin Pie Mix, Canned	½ cup	3	4	0
Winter Squash, All Varieties, Baked, Mashed	2/3 cup	1	1	0
Tofu	½ cup	2	0	2
Hummus	½ cup	4	2	4
POTATOES				
Sweet or Yam	¾ cup	2	3	0
Orange Glazed Yams	¼ cup	3	3	1
Scalloped	½ cup	2	2	1
Mashed	2/3 cup	3	3	2
Au Gratin	½ cup	3	2	3
French Fried, Hashed Brown	½ cup	3	2	4
Baked	1	5	5	7

About the Author

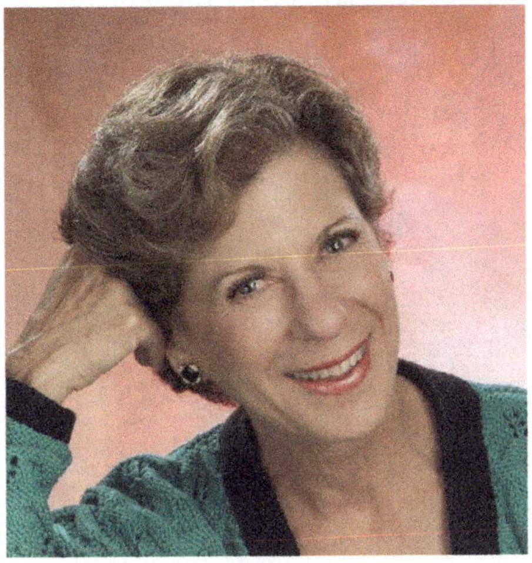

Roberta is an RDN — a registered dietitian nutritionist. She did her undergraduate work at the University of California at Berkeley. She received her master's degree in Nutrition from the University of Washington, followed by her certification and RDN credentials from the Academy of Nutrition and Dietetics. Soon after she became a certified practitioner of the MBTI®.

Roberta is the holder of a U.S. patent for the innovative nutrient monitoring system found in this book, *Drawing the Line on Calories, Carbs, and Fat.* Through research and testing of this system at the University of Washington, she found this connect-the-dots approach to have a statistically significant effect in helping people make healthy changes to their lifestyle habits. She is hoping it will do the same for you.

Roberta also brings something unique to the dietetic profession – she is an expert in the MBTI® (Myers-Briggs Type Indicator® - personality typing). She has combined nutrition and type to present a personality approach to health. Roberta likes to say "know your type and you can improve your life". The way you change your habits should be comfortable with your type. Some of her most recent books include *Health Hijackers, Your Personality Diet,* and *Is It Worth It?* Check them out at www.advantagediets.com or Amazon to find the best way to make healthy decisions, how best to eat according to your type, and how to destress by finding what's essential in your life.

She has written many books, magazine articles, and newspaper columns. She is internationally recognized for her work in nutrition and personality type. Roberta has appeared on television and radio. At heart, she is a teacher no matter whether it's speaking to a group of people, in front of a classroom, or sharing her knowledge in her books.

Roberta and her husband, Larry, started the company, Affordable Editing Services at www.affordableeditingservices.com to help others achieve their dream of having their work published, whether it be a book, blog posts, magazine articles, etc. As they like to say, "no author should be without an editor and coach".

You can find her on Facebook, Twitter and LinkedIn.

Made in the USA
Monee, IL
02 November 2026

67384724R00077